The Complete Guide for Somatic Therapy

How to Relieve Stress, Heal from Trauma, and Strengthen Your Mind-Body Connection

By

Elea Vandez

Guide for somatic therapy

Copyright © 2023, by Elea Vandez

All rights reserved. No part of this publication may be reproduced, distributed, or transmitted in any form or by any means, including photocopying, recording, or other electronic or mechanical methods, without the prior written permission of the publisher, except in the case of brief quotations embodied in critical reviews and certain other noncommercial uses permitted by copyright law.

The information contained in this book is for general informational purposes only. It is not intended as a substitute for professional advice or treatment. The author and publisher disclaim any liability or responsibility for any loss or damage incurred as a result of the use of the information presented in this book.

Guide for somatic therapy

Readers are advised to seek the guidance of qualified professionals or practitioners regarding individual health, mental health, or therapeutic needs. Any reliance on the information within this book is at the reader's discretion and risk.

While every effort has been made to ensure the accuracy of the information provided, the author and publisher make no representations or warranties regarding the completeness, suitability, or reliability of the content.

Guide for somatic therapy

TABLE OF CONTENT

Guide for somatic therapy

Guide for somatic therapy

INTRODUCTION

Welcome to this quest of healing and self-discovery where you may use the power of your body as a compass to navigate the challenges presented by life's events. The concepts of Somatic Therapy shine as a light of hope and transformation in a world where trauma, stress, and the weight of daily pressures may cause us to feel cut off from ourselves.

Imagine times in your life when worry causes your heart to race, when memories cause an aching in your stomach, or when stress causes your chest to constrict. Everybody has experienced this: fighting feelings that appear to overwhelm them and leave us looking for a way out, a route to completeness and calm.

This book is proof that everyone of us has the capacity to not just survive but also

Guide for somatic therapy

flourish. It involves removing the complex webs of stress, trauma, and alienation that have permeated our bodies and brains. Above all, it's about providing you with a road map and a guide to help you uncover the healing and natural wisdom that are already within you.

Somatic therapy is a very human and relevant method to healing, not simply another academic framework. It recognizes that the narrative of our experiences, whether happy and sad, are stored in our bodies. It acknowledges that stress and trauma are physical manifestations of mental emotions as well.

You will come across ideas and methods that, although they may seem familiar, may be incredibly transforming as you go on this journey. Somatic therapy is about recovering what is already yours the intrinsic capacity for self-healing, self-soothing, and

Guide for somatic therapy

self-reconnection rather than piling additional tasks onto your to-do list.

You'll discover basic yet significant routines and activities to help you develop a closer bond with your body and mind.

You own this trip. It's an invitation to deepen your relationship with yourself, to appreciate the knowledge that your body has to offer, and to pay attention to the whispers and yells it makes. It's about establishing a sanctuary inside, where tension melts away like morning mist in the sun, where self-soothing becomes an art form, where healing becomes a way of being rather than a destination.

Allow this book to serve as your guide, a friend, and haven. Let it be an environment that embraces vulnerability, fosters understanding-based growth, and allows the

Guide for somatic therapy

subtleties of your body and mind to work in unison.

Recall this as we work through these pages together: you are not traveling alone. There is a large group of people who are learning, growing, and healing with you. Your bravery and resiliency are demonstrated by every action you take to comprehend the language of your body, every time you embrace the power of your breath, and every time you show self-compassion.

Thus, inhale deeply, let these teachings sink in, and let the path to healing and wholeness to start. The knowledge contained in these chapters is the lighthouse that illuminates the way ahead; you are in possession of the key.

Guide for somatic therapy

Understanding Somatic Therapy.

It's similar to learning your body's hidden language. You know those moments when you're under a lot of stress and all of a sudden your heart is racing, your stomach turns, and your body feels tense? According to somatic therapy, your body is communicating with you and attempting to tell you something significant through those bodily experiences.

It's similar to learning how to decipher these signals and comprehend English sentences. In fact, your body sends signals about your mental state and the ways in which you may still be impacted by the past.

The exciting element, though, is that somatic therapy isn't just for difficult issues. It's also about realizing how resilient and

Guide for somatic therapy

healable your body is. You can really assist your body in releasing tension and stress by doing basic exercises like breathing techniques, certain movements, or mindfulness. It's like pressing a tiny reset button on your body!

Entering Somatic Therapy essentially means embarking on a quest to rediscover your body as your own private sanctuary. You may experiment with feeling healthier and more balanced in your daily life in a safe environment.

This method shows you that feeling happy both physically and emotionally depends on your body, which is more than just a container. It all comes down to paying attention to what your body is telling you, processing the information, and applying it to your life to make you feel better and more relaxed.

Guide for somatic therapy

Somatic therapy is like a road plan that helps you get back to feeling more alive and connected to your body if you've ever been overwhelmed by prior experiences or cut off from it. It's a call to embrace the amazing ability to heal and thrive within you, to be gentle to yourself, and to listen to what your body is telling you.

Chapter 1

What Is Somatic Therapy?

Therapies focused on the mind-body link are grouped together under the heading of somatic psychotherapy. The definition of "somatic" is "pertaining to the body."

Somatic therapy can assist you in releasing any repressed trauma that has gotten "trapped" in your body via the use of certain procedures.

A method to recovery known as somatic therapy acknowledges the influence of trauma, emotions, and prior experiences on the physical body and focuses on the relationship between the mind and body. It recognizes that the events of our lives are

Guide for somatic therapy

imprinted on our bodies, and that we may examine and resolve emotional and psychological problems by being aware of our body's sensations, motions, and postures.

In this treatment, experiencing and comprehending the body's feelings, motions, and patterns takes precedence over merely talking. People can learn more about their emotions and inner experiences by increasing their awareness of these bodily sensations and learning how to interpret them.

In order to assist people in releasing tension, trauma, and stress that has been held in their bodies, somatic therapy combines a number of modalities, including mindfulness, breathwork, body awareness, movement, and touch. These techniques are meant to help one develop a stronger sense of self-awareness, encourage

Guide for somatic therapy

self-control, and support psychological and emotional recovery.

Restoring harmony and integration between the mind and body is the ultimate aim of somatic therapy, which enables people to process traumatic events, live more completely in the present, manage stress, and cultivate better relationships with others and themselves.
Somatic psychology, a body-focused branch of psychology, is the foundation of somatic treatment. The way somatic treatments function is by addressing the ongoing feedback loop that exists between the body and the mind.

Typical psychotherapy (talk therapy) is not the same as somatic therapy. In standard psychotherapy, the therapist just works with the patient's thinking. The body serves as the cornerstone for healing in somatic therapy.

Guide for somatic therapy

Somatic therapists hold that an individual's unpleasant emotions, such as those derived from a traumatic experience, might remain trapped inside the body.

These unpleasant feelings might develop into psychiatric diseases or physical issues like neck or back pain if they are not let go of in a timely manner. People with post-traumatic stress disorder (PTSD) are frequently diagnosed with chronic pain, according to a reliable source.

Somatic therapists employ mind-body methods to help you let go of the stress that is negatively impacting your physical and mental health. Breathing exercises, meditation, dancing, and other physical activities might be included into these strategies.

Guide for somatic therapy

Fundamentals of somatic therapy

Somatic therapy is based on a number of fundamental ideas that influence how it approaches recovery and wellbeing:

Embodied Experience: A key component of somatic therapy is the realization that our bodies hold memories of our experiences in addition to our thoughts. It acknowledges the interdependence of mental, emotional, and physical experiences and the idea that treating one might affect the others.

One of the first steps in learning to release tension from the body is developing body

Guide for somatic therapy

awareness. In addition to learning how to quiet thoughts and feelings, the client also learns to detect and identify body tense spots.

Mind-Body Connection: This therapeutic approach honors and investigates the complex interplay between the mind and body. It acknowledges the relationship between psychological moods and physical health. It strives to improve mental and emotional well-being by paying attention to physical sensations, movements, and postures.

Establishing a strong connection with your body and the soil is known as grounding. Sensing your body, feeling your feet on the ground, and lowering your stress level are all part of grounding.

Guide for somatic therapy

Pendulation: This therapeutic approach takes you from a calm condition to one that is analogous to your traumatic event. You may let go of the stored up energy by doing this multiple times. As the energy is released, you can experience uneasiness or nervousness. You'll be led back to a calm condition each time. You will eventually have the ability to relax on your own.

Titration: Using this method, the therapist walks you through a painful recollection. As you explain the recollection, you will be asked to note any physical changes that occur. The therapist will assist you in addressing any bodily sensations as they arise.

Sequencing is the process of closely observing the sequence in which tense physical feelings depart your body. For example, you may experience a constriction in your throat followed by a constriction in

Guide for somatic therapy

your chest. Then, when the stress departs your body, you can experience shaking.

Resourcing: This is thinking back on the things in your life that provide you a sense of security, such as your connections, your strongest traits, or even a special place you've visited on vacation. It might consist of anything that soothes you. The positive emotions and experiences connected to your resources then come back to you, providing an emotional anchor.

An Approach Informed by Trauma: Somatic Therapy recognizes the effects of trauma on the body and mind. It aims to treat trauma by using both talk therapy and physical methods, enabling people to safely process and let go of terrible memories that have been held in their bodies.

Nonverbal Communication: It acknowledges that body language,

Guide for somatic therapy

gestures, and physical clues make up a large portion of nonverbal communication. These nonverbal cues are used in somatic therapy in order to identify and treat underlying psychological and emotional conditions.

Integration and Regulation: The goal of somatic therapy is to promote mental and physical integration. In order to assist people manage stress, control their emotions, and regain balance, it places a strong emphasis on self-regulation strategies including movement, breathwork, and mindfulness exercises.

Holistic Healing: Somatic Therapy strives for holistic healing, taking into account the body, mind, and soul of the patient, as opposed to only treating symptoms. It fosters a greater sense of completeness and wellbeing by encouraging people to

Guide for somatic therapy

consider their experiences in the perspective of their full being.

Evolution and History

The origins and development of somatic therapy may be found in a variety of fields and traditions that acknowledged the close relationship between the body and the mind.

Early Impacts

Ancient Eastern disciplines that emphasize the integration of body, mind, and spirit for well-being, such as yoga, tai chi, and meditation, are the origins of somatic therapy. These exercises emphasized the role that movement, breathing, and body sensations have in developing consciousness and inner peace.

Guide for somatic therapy

Body-Centered Methods

Body-oriented psychotherapy benefited greatly from the contributions of individuals such as Wilhelm Reich and Alexander Lowen in the early to mid-20th century. Reich's work with physical tension release and character structure has informed our knowledge of how emotions show themselves in the body. Lowen investigated the connection between physical posture and emotional expressiveness using bioenergetics.

Development of Somatic Experiencing

Somatic Experiencing was developed in part because of the groundbreaking work of
Guide for somatic therapy

Dr. Peter Levine in the late 20th century. Based on his studies of how trauma is naturally released from animals, Levine developed methods to assist people in removing traumatic stress from their bodies. The goal of somatic experiencing is to enhance the body's natural healing ability and reframe trauma via physical sensations.

Somatic therapy was included into a number of psychotherapy techniques over time. Experts in disciplines like psychology, counseling, and bodywork started using somatic approaches in their work after realizing the benefits of treating the body in addition to the mind through conventional talk therapy.

The growth of Somatic Therapy was further aided by the increasing acceptance of embodiment techniques and mindfulness-based therapies. The acceptance of mindfulness-focused

Guide for somatic therapy

techniques, breathwork, body scan exercises, and movement-based treatments increased, contributing to a deeper comprehension of the mind-body relationship.

Acknowledgment in the Treatment of Trauma:

The use of Somatic Therapy in the treatment of trauma has grown significantly. As the understanding of how trauma is stored in the body grew, so did the value of somatic therapies in trauma recovery for therapists and researchers. Somatic components were also incorporated into trauma-focused treatment through methods like EMDR (Eye Movement Desensitization and Reprocessing).

With an increasing amount of evidence demonstrating its effectiveness in treating chronic pain, mental health issues,

Guide for somatic therapy

stress-related diseases, and trauma, somatic therapy is still developing today. It includes a variety of methods that emphasize the role of the body in healing and self-discovery, such as Hakomi Therapy, Sensorimotor Psychotherapy, and Somatic Experiencing.

This evolutionary path represents an increasing recognition of the body-mind connection and the need of incorporating the body's wisdom and feelings into therapeutic interventions for overall healing and wellbeing.

Guide for somatic therapy

Chapter 2

The Mind-Body Connection

The concept of the mind-body link is by no means new. The mind and body were considered as one unit in almost every medical system in the world until around 300 years ago. However, the Western culture began to view the mind and body as two separate things from the 17th century. According to this perspective, the body was completely disconnected from the consciousness and resembled a machine with interchangeable, autonomous parts.

There were undoubtedly advantages to this Western perspective, which laid the groundwork for advancements in allopathic medicine, including surgery, trauma treatment, and medications. But it also minimized humankind's intrinsic capacity for healing and drastically curtailed scientific research into the emotional and spiritual lives of people.

Over the course of the 20th century, this perspective began to shift. Scholars started investigating the correlation between the mind and body, presenting intricate connections between the two through scientific means.

Understanding the Integral Connection

The feedback loop between your body and mind is how the mind-body link operates.

Guide for somatic therapy

Your thoughts are influenced by your feelings and vice versa. Your thoughts and feelings can communicate with each other through the mind-body link.

The term "feeling" suggests a bodily experience, even if you could conceive of your feelings as something that just exists in your head. Your emotions are physical sensations. Your emotions are all defined by physical experiences.

For instance, you may have anxiety in your abdomen. Your heart rate may increase. As you try to defend yourself, your posture may go from open to closed.

You may feel at ease and proud of yourself when you are confident. You have control over your heart rate and breathing. You may have a powerful, serene feeling. Your feelings will influence your ideas.

Guide for somatic therapy

Realizing how our body and spirit are connected is similar to appreciating the friendship between two closest friends who finish each other's sentences. It's about realizing that although they are distinct entities, they are intricately entwined and positively support and influence one another.

Consider your body as your physical home and the means of transportation through life. It's your reflection in the mirror, your gait, and your perception of the world as your own little spacecraft on this adventure we call life.

Imagine your soul as your inner voice, your true self, the part of you that dreams, experiences emotions, and connects with something more than yourself. This is your soul. It steers your ideas, ideals, and beliefs, acting as your inner cheerleader.

Guide for somatic therapy

The catch is that one's actions have an impact on the other. Your thoughts and feelings might be affected when your body feels pressured or exhausted. Similarly, bodily strain or tiredness may manifest as spiritual or emotional fatigue or overload.

The secret sauce? bringing these two partners together in harmony. It's similar to finding the ideal beat in a dance when your body, mind, and spirit are all in harmony. You have a sense of wholeness, vibrancy, and awareness of both the outside world and oneself.

It seems sense that when one is out of balance, the other would also feel a little off.

Consider it like an orchestra: for a stunning symphony of wellbeing, you want every instrument to perform in unison.

Guide for somatic therapy

This is where things get interesting! Your body and spirit are linked via a variety of disciplines such as yoga, meditation, prayer, and simply taking a stroll in the outdoors. They promote balance and serenity by assisting you in making a connection with your inner self.

This connection relates to health as well as happiness. Many people think that emotional or spiritual imbalances can affect our physical health and vice versa. Hence, taking care of this relationship is similar to taking care of a garden; when you take care of one plant, the entire area grows.

In the end, it's a personal journey to uncover your experiences, values, and convictions. Having a greater knowledge of this connection gives you the ability to negotiate life's ups and downs with inner calm, compassion for others, and a better understanding of yourself.

Guide for somatic therapy

Accepting this link between body and soul is the first step in a path of self-discovery, healing, and immense love for the amazing creature that is you. It also marks the beginning of a greater knowledge of the world and yourself.

Impact on Trauma Healing

The link between the mind and body is quite potent. The body and mind are meant to function together as allies to promote the best possible physical and mental well-being. However, there are instances when they are antagonistic. The mind-body link may be difficult, much like most partnerships.

Guide for somatic therapy

Our biological functioning can be positively or adversely impacted by our memories, ideas, feelings, and attitudes. Put another way, there is a clear correlation between our mental and physical well-being. Our mental health may be favorably or negatively impacted by our physical well-being, which includes our diet, exercise routine, sleep patterns, and alcohol and drug usage. Furthermore, it is easier to initiate the fight-or-flight response in young adults due to the brain's immaturity.

A disconnection between the mind and body might occasionally feel like an unforeseen shock caused by a bodily experience, such as smelling or hearing something that brings back a distressing memory. Alternatively, it may seem as though you're viewing yourself from the perspective of someone else. This is almost often a response to anything that

Guide for somatic therapy

the subconscious found to be too much or too unpleasant.

In order to combat the perceived threat to one's safety, the body's "fight or flight" reaction is initiated, resulting in a surge of stress hormones that cause physiological changes. The heart and breathing rates quicken, and muscles stiffen. Repetitive stimulation of this stress response wears down the body over time.

A young adult's body will remember if they had emotional, physical, or sexual abuse as a child or adolescent, despite their best efforts to forget. Thus, among many other symptoms, the repressed memories may cause headaches, backaches, clenched jaws, flashbacks, nightmares, nervous thoughts, and so on.

It's like opening a door to your inner sanctuary, a secure place where scars may

Guide for somatic therapy

be healed and resilience can grow when trauma is healed via the body-soul connection. Trauma frequently has a tremendous effect on the body, spirit, and mind in addition to the mind. Comprehending this connection becomes essential in the healing process.

Stored in the Body: Long after the traumatic incident has gone, physical feelings, tension, or pain may still be present in the body due to stored trauma. These feelings frequently serve as signals, bringing up memories of the event and evoking strong emotions.

Impact on the Mind and Emotions: Trauma has a profound effect on one's mental and emotional health. It might result in depressive, anxious, or tense sensations all the time. It may also have an impact on our views of the world, other people, and ourselves.

Guide for somatic therapy

Disconnection from the Self: Witnessing trauma can cause a person to feel cut off from their body and spirit. It might resemble being caught in a painful loop or having a sense of alienation from both oneself and other people.

The Body as Messenger: Understanding how the body stores trauma is essential to the healing process. Sensations from the body, such as constriction, a fast heartbeat, or shallow breathing, might serve as messengers or indicators of unresolved trauma.

Guide for somatic therapy

The Function of Somatic Therapy

Methods such as Somatic Therapy are essential for the healing of trauma. They assist people in processing emotions and memories that are held in the body by reestablishing a connection with physical sensations as a means of treating trauma.

Empowerment via Awareness: People may reclaim control of their lives by learning more about the physical and psychological effects of trauma. Along with learning how to identify triggers, they also acquire skills in self-control and managing intense emotions.

Integration and Healing: Somatic Therapy methods, such breathing exercises, grounding exercises, or gentle movement, assist in releasing the body's

Guide for somatic therapy

accumulated stress and trauma. This procedure fosters healing, empowerment, and a sense of safety.

Restoring Balance: Finding one's own path back to equilibrium, reestablishing trust, and recovering a sense of security and completeness are all important aspects of healing trauma through the body-soul connection. Discovering harmony between the body, mind, and spirit is similar to assembling a jigsaw.

Embracing Resilience: In the end, this healing process is also about accepting resilience, which is everyone's natural ability to recover, develop, and flourish in spite of adversity.

Guide for somatic therapy

Chapter 3

Developing Somatic Awareness

To become somatically aware, one must have a profound comprehension of and connection to one's physical experiences, movements, and sensations. The basis of somatic therapy and other mind-body techniques is somatic awareness, which enables people to successfully identify, understand, and respond to bodily sensations and emotions. This is a thorough examination of growing somatic awareness:

1. An Introduction to Somatic Awareness:

The Body-Mind Connection: Somatic awareness emphasizes the close

Guide for somatic therapy

connection between the body and mind, emphasizing the ways in which physical experiences impact feelings, ideas, and actions.

Observing Feelings:It entails being perceptive to physical cues, free from bias or interpretation, such as tenseness, ease, warmth, tingling, pain, or pleasure.

2. Methods for Building Somatic Awareness:

Mindfulness Exercises:Focusing on body sensations through mindful movement, body scans, or mindfulness meditation helps cultivate present-moment awareness.

Breathwork: Making use of breathwork exercises helps cultivate an understanding of how various breathing patterns impact physical and mental conditions.

3. Body Scan and Progressive Muscle Relaxation:

Guide for somatic therapy

Body Scan:is a mental scan of the body's various sections, noting any tensions, feelings, or comfortable spots. It helps one gain insight into the body's reactions.

Progressive Muscle Relaxation (PMR):By systematically tensing and releasing specific muscle groups, one can increase awareness of tension and relaxation in the body.

4. **Grounding Through the Senses**: **Activating the Senses:** Grounding activities that include taste, smell, sight, sound, or touch can anchor people to the present moment and promote bodily awareness.

Method:

5-4-3-2-1 To improve sensory awareness, this approach asks participants to identify five things they can see, four things they can touch, three things they can hear, two things they can smell, and one item they can taste.

Guide for somatic therapy

5.   **Body-Centered   Practices   and Movement:**

Yoga, Tai Chi, or Qigong: Practicing movement-based arts promotes awareness of physical sensations and deepens the link between movement and emotions.

Dance therapy: This approach uses dance to investigate how the body expresses emotions and helps identify and manage feelings via movement.

6.   **Emotion   Tracking   and   Somatic Experiencing**:

Somatic Experiencing (SE): Methods in SE entail monitoring physical sensations associated with feelings in order to facilitate comprehension and processing of emotional memories held inside the body.

Emotion tracking: Identifying relationships between body sensations and emotions is

Guide for somatic therapy

improved by noting and labeling emotions together with related feelings.

7. **Journaling and Reflective Practices:** - **Body-Mind Journals**: Writing about one's physical experiences, feelings, or movements encourages introspection and a deeper comprehension of one's own body's reactions to feelings or circumstances.
Self-Reflection: Regular self-reflection promotes awareness of the mind-body link and facilitates the identification of triggers and patterns.

8. Approaches Informed by Trauma:
Examining Trauma Reactions: Somatic awareness practices support the identification and management of physical reactions to traumatic experiences in the past, which promotes healing and trauma resolution.
Controlling Stress Reactions: Gaining knowledge about how the body responds to

Guide for somatic therapy

stress encourages self-control and stress-reduction.

Somatic awareness development is a continuous process that includes developing mindfulness, strengthening the connection with physical sensations, and learning to read your body's signs. People can better understand their emotional states, enhance self-regulation, and promote general well-being by developing this awareness. Developing and honing somatic awareness abilities can be facilitated by consulting with a somatic therapist or by engaging in regular somatic practices.

Embodied practices of healing

Using the body as a main instrument for processing, integrating, and overcoming emotional, psychological, and physical

Guide for somatic therapy

discomfort is known as embodied healing methods. These methods emphasize the significance of physiological experiences in the healing process and acknowledge the interdependence of the mind, body, and spirit. This is a thorough examination of embodied healing practices:

1.**Resolving Trauma with Somatic Therapy:**

Somatic Experiencing (SE): Methods center on physical experiences to help release trauma that has been held in the body, enabling the body to finish its halted fight-or-flight reaction and promoting healing.

Trauma-Informed Bodywork: Using body-centered techniques to treat trauma, this method supports the release of tension that has been held and fosters healing from traumatic experiences in the past.

Guide for somatic therapy

2. Methods of Mind-Body Integration:

Mindfulness-Based Stress Reduction (MBSR): This technique lowers stress and promotes healing by cultivating awareness of one's own body's sensations, thoughts, and emotions.

Body-Mind Centering: A method to healing and self-discovery that examines the anatomy, movement, and consciousness of the body.

3. Treatments Based on Movement:

Yoga therapy: This approach uses a combination of breathing exercises, physical postures, and mindfulness to ease tension, promote emotional healing, and relieve stress.

Using dance and movement as a means of self-expression and emotional processing, dance movement therapy helps people

Guide for somatic therapy

release their feelings and heal from traumatic experiences.

4. Relaxation and Breathwork Methods:

Breath Awareness: Techniques such as mindful breathing or pranayama help people relax, feel less anxious, and manage their emotions and heal.

- **Progressive Muscle Relaxation (PMR):** This technique involves methodically tensing and releasing muscle groups to ease physical tension, encourage relaxation, and support general healing.

5. Expressive Arts Therapies: Art therapy is a non-verbal and symbolic way to process trauma, explore emotions, and promote healing via creative expression through a variety of art genres.

Music Therapy: Using rhythm, melody, and lyrics, music may help people express their emotions, lower stress levels, and aid in healing.

Guide for somatic therapy

6. **Mindful Movement and Body Awareness:**

Tai Chi or Qigong: Using mindful breathing and slow, purposeful motions to improve body-mind awareness and encourage healing.

Sensory Awareness Techniques:Promoting increased awareness and self-regulation by encouraging people to observe their physical experiences without passing judgment.

7. **Touch-Based recovery Modalities**:

- **Massage Therapy:** Applying touch to ease tension in the body, lower stress levels, and enhance emotional stability can help with both emotional and physical recovery.

-**Acupuncture or Acupressure:**Stimulating certain areas of the body to ease physical

Guide for somatic therapy

discomfort, reduce stress, and promote holistic healing.

8.. Embodied Psychotherapy and EMDR: Sensorimotor Psychotherapy:Combining talk therapy with somatic approaches to treat emotional problems held in the body, this approach promotes healing and emotional control.

Traumatic events that have been stored in the body can be processed and healed with the use of bilateral stimulation in Eye Movement Desensitization and Reprocessing (EMDR).

9. Self-Compassion and Inner Resourcing:

Self-Soothing Practices: Practicing self-care techniques that cultivate self-compassion and aid in healing, such as self-massage, visualization, or relaxation techniques.

Guide for somatic therapy

Inner Resourcing: Creating safe havens, constructive self-narratives, and internal resources to promote resilience and healing under trying circumstances.

Holistic and varied methods are provided by embodied healing techniques, which acknowledge the mind-body connection during the healing process. Through the development of self-awareness, emotional control, and trauma resolution, these methods assist people in their quest for complete healing and general wellbeing. Tailored therapies to help the healing process can be obtained by seeking guidance from therapists or trained practitioners knowledgeable in embodied healing techniques.

Guide for somatic therapy

Chapter 4

Neurobiology of Trauma

The study of neurobiology focuses on the nervous system and the functioning of the brain. The field investigates the functioning of the nervous system, the brain, and other structures including the spinal cord. Physiology and neuroscience are subsets of neurobiology.
Researchers that specialize in neurobiology examine how the nerve system and brain work.

The prefrontal cortex is the area of the brain that makes decisions and choices; it is in charge of logical reasoning, organizing well-thought-out actions, retaining crucial details, etc. A person's "Fear Circuitry" may

Guide for somatic therapy

activate during a traumatic experience or when they are experiencing intense fear, which causes the prefrontal brain to start functioning less efficiently. This implies that a person experiencing trauma might not be able to reason Their brain is in survival mode and the fear circuitry is completely avoiding their prefrontal cortex, therefore it is not a question of choice.

While most people understand the idea of "fight or flight," study reveals that there is also a third reaction known as "freeze." A deer in headlights is a classic illustration of this fear response in humans; in fact, freezing, as opposed to fighting back or fleeing, is the most common response to trauma or terror.

Some survivors may also have strong survival reactions like collapsed immobility or tonic immobility in addition to freezing. If you have ever witnessed a terrified possum

Guide for somatic therapy

go limp, you are aware of this brain response. Survival tactics such as being limp, feeling "sleepy" or passing out, or being totally immobile or mute are hardwired into our brains; even apex predators like sharks have similar reactions! It's not a decision the individual is making, nor is it an indication of weakness.

Moreover, dissociation, a survival reflex, that causes a person to feel detached from their body or to switch to "auto-pilot" may occur in survivors. When someone is in auto-pilot mode, they are depending on habitual patterns of being rather than employing their prefrontal brain to make judgments. Habitual reactions stem from socialization; women, for instance, are conditioned to be kind and agreeable in order to "save face" or appease. This implies that even if a person may act sexually, say nice things, or even smile during an attack, they are not really giving their permission; rather, they are feeling intense anxiety and their brain is reacting instinctively as a survival mechanism.

Following a distressing incident, memories are encoded differently. The "fear circuitry" in the brain directs attention to certain aspects during the attack, and these facts are more likely to be stored into memory than peripheral details. The brain does not register memories in chronological order, and there are gaps in memory. For instance, a victim could remember the perpetrator's cologne scent rather well, but they might not remember the exact appearance of the room. Time-sequence information, such as the order in which sexual activities happened, and contextual information, such as the arrangement of a room, are frequently stored poorly. Again, this is a frequent effect on the brain when the "fear circuitry" survival reaction kicks in;

Guide for somatic therapy

it is not a deliberate decision made by a survivor about what to focus on or recall after an assault.

Gaining insight into the neurobiology of trauma is akin to delving into the inner workings of our bodies and minds during traumatic events. It's about figuring out how our nervous system and brain react to difficult situations and how these reactions affect our feelings, actions, and general well-being.

Upon experiencing trauma, our brain's alert system malfunctions. Think of it as our amygdala, the area of the brain in charge of emotions and survival instincts, going into overdrive when we hear a loud fire alarm. Stress chemicals like cortisol and adrenaline are released as a result, preparing our bodies to fight, run, or freeze in the event of danger.

Guide for somatic therapy

This is when the exciting part starts. Trauma changes our brains in more ways than just how we feel. Consider the several brain regions working together to manage a storm's aftermath. When the amygdala becomes overactive, we experience jitteriness, anxiety, or overwhelming terror. The memory-related hippocampus may find it difficult to piece together a consistent account of what transpired. Furthermore, intense emotions may be difficult for the brain's decision-making region, the prefrontal cortex, to control.

Our stress response system might become unbalanced after prolonged exposure to trauma. It seems like you're perpetually on high alert, constantly scanning the horizon for threats, even in circumstances that appear secure. Constant stress may lead to mental health problems like anxiety, sadness, or post-traumatic stress disorder

Guide for somatic therapy

(PTSD), as well as problems with our focus, sleep, and even physical health.

The bright side is that our brain's incredible neuroplasticity is a blessing. It's how the brain adjusts and rewires itself. Following trauma, the brain may recover and rearrange itself with the support of therapies and practices that capitalize on this, such as mindfulness and somatic therapy.

Managing emotions is only one aspect of effective trauma healing; another is acknowledging and promoting the alterations in our brains. Body-focused therapies, such as breathing exercises or light physical activities, try to help relax the body, control the nervous system's reaction, and allow the brain to recuperate.

In this path, developing resilience is essential. It's similar to giving our bodies and minds an additional push. Restoring

Guide for somatic therapy

balance and resilience in the face of trauma is mostly dependent on developing social relationships, learning good coping mechanisms, and creating a sense of safety.

Therefore, comprehending the neurobiology of trauma is like figuring out the complex language that both our bodies and minds speak. It clarifies the impact of trauma on us and points us in the direction of practices and treatments that promote healing, transform our brains, and enable us to overcome the most difficult obstacles in life with more strength.

The Brain Reactions to Trauma and Stress

Now let's explore the many ways in which the brain reacts to stress and trauma:

Guide for somatic therapy

The brain's "alarm system," the amygdala, activates in response to stressful or traumatic events. This is known as the amygdala's reaction. It quickly scans the environment to determine whether something is dangerous. This examination sets off the body's stress reaction and elicits an instantaneous emotional response, often feelings of dread or worry.

Hormonal Cascade - HPA Axis: The Hypothalamic-Pituitary-Adrenal (HPA) axis is composed of the pituitary, adrenal, and hypothalamus. The pituitary gland produces adrenocorticotropic hormone (ACTH) in reaction to stress or trauma by directing the brain to release corticotropin-releasing hormone (CRH). Stress hormones like cortisol and adrenaline are then released into the bloodstream by the adrenal glands in response to an ACTH signal.

Guide for somatic therapy

Physiological Alterations: The body is overflowed with stress hormones, which cause a series of physiological adjustments. Blood pressure rises, respiration quickens, muscles stiffen, and heart rate accelerates. These physiological shifts prime the body for rapid response to perceived threats, preparing it for either the fight-or-flight or freeze response.

Impact on Memory: Trauma and stress have an effect on how memories are processed. It may be difficult for the hippocampus, which is in charge of creating and preserving memories, to encode the traumatic event into comprehensible memories. This might lead to gaps in memory or fragmented, intrusive recollections, which can make it difficult to fully recall the event's specifics.

Impairment of the Prefrontal Cortex: Under stress or trauma, the prefrontal

Guide for somatic therapy

cortex, which is involved in problem-solving, decision-making, emotional regulation, and social behavior moderation, may become impaired. This region may find it difficult to control strong emotions, which might make it difficult to efficiently digest information, control impulses, or manage emotions.

Neuroplasticity and Changes: Prolonged stress or trauma exposure can physically change the structure and function of the brain. The brain's ability to rearrange and change in response to events is known as neuroplasticity. Depending on the severity and kind of the trauma, this adaptation may make recovery more difficult or easier.

Effects of persistent Stress: Over time, the brain and nervous system may adjust to persistent activation brought on by stress or trauma. Even in safe situations, this can lead to a continuous state of heightened arousal, where people are always on high

Guide for somatic therapy

alert. This ongoing stress reaction can exacerbate physical health conditions like compromised immune systems or cardiovascular difficulties as well as mental health conditions like anxiety and despair.

Knowing these intricate brain reactions to stress and trauma can help people better understand the vast range of emotional, mental, and physical symptoms people may encounter. The goal of therapeutic interventions and practices is to control these reactions in people who have experienced stress or trauma in order to aid in healing, restore equilibrium, and build resilience.

Guide for somatic therapy

Chapter 5

Stress-Reduction and Self-Soothing Methods

Deep breathing exercises

Deep breathing can assist in nervous system calmness. In order to promote relaxation and lower tension, methods such as diaphragmatic breathing or box breathing include taking a deep breath, holding it for a little while, and then gently expelling.

Exercises involving deep breathing are effective methods for relaxing the mind, lowering tension, and encouraging sleep. Here's a more thorough examination of many deep breathing methods:

1. **Diaphragmatic breathing:** this is also known as belly breathing, is a method that involves using the diaphragm, the muscle

Guide for somatic therapy

that separates the abdomen and the chest. For diaphragmatic breathing exercises:

- Either take a seat comfortably or rest flat on your back.

- Put your hands on your abdomen and your chest, respectively.

- Take a deep breath through your nostrils, raising your abdomen (visualize filling it with air).

- Let your tummy drop as you gently exhale through your lips.

- Feel the hand on your belly rise and fall while the hand on your chest stays relatively static as you breathe in and out. Concentrate on extending your abdomen.

- Continue in a slow, rhythmic manner for a few breaths.

2. **4-7-8 Breathing (Relaxing Breath):** This method has precise counts for taking a breath, holding it, and letting it out.

- Take a four-second breath through your nose.

Guide for somatic therapy

- Breathe out slowly for seven seconds.

- Let out the breath gently through your lips for eight seconds.

- Continue in this manner for more rounds, keeping your beat constant.

3. **Box Breathing (Square Breathing):** This technique forms a square by inhaling, holding, expelling, and then holding again at equal counts.

Take a four-second deep breath through your nose.

Hold your breath,for four counts,

Let out a slow, four-second breath through your mouth.

Hold your breath for a further four seconds.

Keep going in this manner, making a "box" pattern, and repeat several times.

4. **Alternate Nostril Breathing (Nadi Shodhana):** This method seeks to promote calmness and mental clarity by balancing the left and right sides of the brain:

Guide for somatic therapy

- Take a comfortable seat and sit up straight.

- Using your thumb to close your right nostril, take a deep breath through your left.

- Completely exhale by closing your left nostril with your ring finger and opening your right nose.

- Breathe in via your right nose.

- Shut your right nose and open your left, fully exhaling.

- Continue in cycles of this alternating pattern.

These kinds of deep breathing exercises assist in triggering the body's relaxation response, which lowers stress hormones and fosters a feeling of peace. Deep breathing exercises on a regular basis can increase lung capacity, oxygen flow, reduce muscular tension, and foster a deeper sensation of relaxation and wellbeing.

Guide for somatic therapy

Meditation and mindfulness:

Mindfulness

Being mindful is being aware of the present moment without passing judgment on it. It's similar to observing your thoughts, emotions, and external environment without labeling them as positive or negative. You might not think about the past or future, instead concentrating on your breathing or your current task.

Meditation: Think of meditation as mental exercise. The fundamental goal is to sit silently and focus, however there are several methods to achieve this. While some meditation techniques concentrate on breathing, others emphasize soothing the mind or even practicing kindness toward oneself and others.

Guide for somatic therapy

Benefits: Reducing stress, improving concentration, and increasing emotional awareness are all possible with mindfulness and meditation. They can also improve your general mood and help you become friendlier to both yourself and other people.

These may be practiced by taking short daily breaks to stop and be aware of your thoughts and feelings, by enrolling in classes or utilizing applications that walk you through it, or by just sitting quietly and focusing on your breathing. These routines have the potential to calm you down and improve your attention and contentment over time.

The progressive muscle relaxation (PMR)

Guide for somatic therapy

A method of fostering relaxation and methodically lowering physical tension is called progressive muscle relaxation, or PMR. It entails tensing and then releasing various muscle groups in your body. For a clearer explanation, see this:

How it works:
1. **Tensing Muscles:** To begin, tense a particular muscle group in your body for a brief period of time, generally five to ten seconds. You could, for instance, tense your shoulders or clench your hands firmly.
2. **Releasing Tension**: Once you have tensed, gradually release the tension while focusing on the sensation of relaxation that arises from the muscles relaxing. It feels like releasing all of the tension and allowing the muscles to expand and become at ease.
3. **Systematic Process**: You repeat the procedure while moving on to the next muscle group. Major muscle groups including the hands, arms, shoulders, face,

Guide for somatic therapy

neck, belly, thighs, and so forth are frequently worked in a certain order.

Why It Works: PMR helps your body distinguish between physical stress and relaxation, which reduces physical tension. It helps your body learn how to relax more efficiently by purposefully tensing and relaxing your muscles.

Calms the Mind: Your body's relaxation might send a message to your mind to follow suit. It may lessen anxiety and tension.

Improves Sleep: By relaxing your body and mind before bed, practicing PMR will help you fall asleep more easily.

Progressive Muscle Relaxation Techniques:

Guide for somatic therapy

1. Look for a Quiet Area: Take a seat or sleep down in a peaceful area where you won't be bothered.

2. Start at One End: You might start with your hands or feet. One muscle group at a time is the focus.
3. Tense and Hold: Without straining or injuring yourself, tense the muscles in that region for five to ten seconds.

4. Release and Relax: Let go of the tension gradually and sense that all of your muscles have relaxed.

5. Move to the Next Muscle Group: Continue the procedure, progressively working your way across your body, using the subsequent muscle group.

Practice Makes Perfect: You'll get better at identifying when your muscles are stiff and knowing how to relax them with repeated

Guide for somatic therapy

attempts. It may take a few tries to get acclimated to the procedure. With time, PMR may be a useful technique for stress management and for encouraging a more laid-back attitude.

Using your mind to conjure up calming, vivid mental images is known as guided imagery or visualization, and it is a technique for relaxation. It's similar to going on a peaceful, mental vacation. For a more thorough explanation, see this:

How it Works:

1. **Create a Calm Scene**: Firstly, look for a peaceful, comfortable spot to sit or lie down. Shut your eyes and visualize a calm, secure haven in your thoughts. It might be any peaceful place that you find soothing, such as a beach, forest, or garden.
2. **Activate Your Senses**: Provide as much information as you can in the situation.

Guide for somatic therapy

Imagine the colors, forms, and environment that you perceive. Incorporate noises such as birds chirping or waves smashing. Sensate the softness of the grass beneath your feet or the warmth of the sun. To enhance the realism and immersion of the images, use all of your senses.

3. **Discover and Savor**: Spend some time exploring this mental haven. Envision yourself strolling around this location and taking in all of its splendor. Take in the scene's peacefulness, take in the nuances, and inhale the fresh air.

4. **Maintain Calm:** While engaging in guided imagery, concentrate on calming your mind and body. Gently return your focus to the serene environment you've created if any distracting ideas arise.

Benefits

Guide for somatic therapy

Stress Reduction: By calming your body and mind, guided imagery eases tension and stress.

Emotional Regulation: By offering a peaceful, mental haven, it can aid in the regulation of emotions.

Increased Concentration and Creativity: By teaching your mind to focus and see vivid details, visualization exercises can help you become more creative, focused, and adept at solving problems.

Enhanced Well-Being: Consistently engaging in guided visualization exercises can enhance one's sense of inner tranquility and general well-being.

How to Use Guided Imagery in Practice:

Guided Sessions: Apps, the internet, and recordings all provide guided imaging

Guide for somatic therapy

sessions in audio format. A narrator leads these sessions, directing your imagination and explaining soothing scenes as they help you visualize.

Self-Guided Imagery: Another option is to write your own screenplay for visualizing. Begin by describing your peaceful location and the feelings, sounds, and experiences you wish to conjure. In a peaceful, calm place, record your script or just walk yourself through the visuals.

Personalization is essential as each person may have a distinct peaceful spot. The secret is to conjure up images that calm you down, make you feel at ease, and promote relaxation. With consistent use, guided imagery can be an effective technique for lowering stress, encouraging calmness, and cultivating relaxation.

Guide for somatic therapy

Body work or self-massage

Using your hands or basic tools to apply pressure, movement, or manipulation to various body regions can help you relax, release tension, and improve your general well-being. This practice is known as self-massage or bodywork. Here's a more thorough investigation:

Self-Massage Techniques:

1. **Using Your Hands**: You can massage tense or uncomfortable regions with your hands. Methods consist of:
Effleurage: To warm up the region, use long, light strokes with your palms or fingertips.
Kneading: Similar to kneading dough, knead and relieve tension in muscles with your fingers or knuckles.

Guide for somatic therapy

Circular Friction. Targeted stress locations with circular movements under hard pressure.

Compression: To relieve tension, gently press your palms or fingers into your muscles.

2.**Self-Massage equipment:**A variety of equipment may be used to help with self-massage:

Foam Rollers: Rolling back and forth on the roller can help you massage major muscular areas like your thighs, calves, and back.

Massage Balls: Little balls that are frequently used on the floor or against walls to target certain spots of stress.

Handheld Massagers: Tools including rollers or knobs for applying pressure to difficult-to-reach regions or those in need of a more thorough massage.

Benefits of Self-Massage:

Guide for somatic therapy

Muscle Relaxation: Self-massage helps alleviate tense, tight muscles and increase suppleness.

Stress Reduction: By encouraging relaxation and lowering stress hormones, it calms the body and reduces stress.

Pain Relief: Applying pressure to strained or painful regions can ease pain and reduce discomfort.

Enhanced Circulation: Light tissue manipulation can improve blood flow, providing muscles with more nutrition and oxygen while also assisting in the elimination of waste.

Self-Massage Techniques:

1. **Find a Quiet Space**: Look for a peaceful, comfortable area where you may unwind without being bothered.

Guide for somatic therapy

2. **Apply little Pressure**: If necessary, apply little pressure at first and then gradually increase it. Refrain from creating discomfort or agony.

3. **Pay Attention to Tension regions**: Concentrate on any painful or tense regions. The neck, shoulders, back, arms, legs, and feet are common locations.

4. **Try Different Techniques**: See which ones work best for you by caressing, kneading, or applying pressure.

5. **Be Mindful**: Observe your body's reaction. Should something cause you pain or discomfort, either modify your method or cease.

Frequent self-massage sessions can be a beneficial addition to your self-care regimen, aiding in your relaxation and well-being

Guide for somatic therapy

while assisting you in decompressing and releasing tense muscles.

Grounding techniques

By keeping you rooted in the here and now, grounding techniques provide you a sense of security and steadiness. They're especially beneficial when you're feeling anxious, stressed, or overwhelmed. Here's a closer examination of grounding methods:

Different Grounding Technique Types:

1. Sensory Grounding:

5-4-3-2-1 technique:Using your senses, take note of:

Guide for somatic therapy

- Five objects that are visible to you.
Four tangible items.
Three audible things.
-Two things you can smell.
- One taste, or concentrate on how your breath feels.

2. **Physical Grounding:**

Deep Breathing: Concentrate on your breathing and sense the air coming into and going out of your body. This relaxes the nervous system and draws focus to the here and now.

Physical Examination: From head to toe, slowly examine your body, noticing any tensions or feelings. As you go, consciously release the tension in every body area.

Mental Grounding:

Counting or Reciting: Count backwards from a big number (e.g., 100) by three-digit

Guide for somatic therapy

intervals, or repeat a well-known poem or song lyrics.

Object Naming: Name and describe everything around you verbally or mentally. This serves to draw attention to the environment.

4. **Visualization grounding**:

Safe Place Imagery: Close your eyes and visualize yourself in a location where you are entirely protected and at ease. Imagine it in full detail, using all of your senses.

How Grounding Techniques help:

- **Anxiety Reduction**: Grounding techniques assist in shifting focus away from unpleasant thoughts or overpowering emotions, therefore lowering anxiety levels.

Guide for somatic therapy

-**Mindfulness Practice**: They promote mindfulness, which allows you to be present and focused on the here and now.

-**Emotional Regulation:** Grounding can assist with emotional regulation by offering a sense of control and stability.

- **Tension Reduction**: Grounding practices can reduce tension and increase relaxation by drawing attention to the present moment.

When to Use Grounding Techniques:
   - When feeling panicked, anxious, or overwhelmed by emotions.
- When you are separated from reality.
- In difficult times, to recover concentration or center yourself.

How to Practice Grounding: Experiment with several ways to see what works best for you.
- Practice often, even when you aren't feeling overwhelmed, to improve your ability

Guide for somatic therapy

to use grounding techniques when necessary.
- Be patient and kind to yourself; it may take some time to find the proper grounding approach for you.

Grounding methods are simple yet powerful strategies to anchor oneself in the present moment, offering a sense of security and peace in the face of stressful or challenging situations.

Aromatherapy

Aromatherapy is a holistic therapeutic approach that promotes well-being, harmony, and relaxation by using natural plant extracts known as essential oils. These concentrated oils are obtained from various plant components, such as flowers, leaves, bark, or roots, and are utilized in a variety of ways to provide medicinal advantages. Here's a more in-depth look:

Guide for somatic therapy

How to Use Essential Oils:

1.**Diffusers**: These gadgets disseminate essential oils into the air, allowing you to breathe in their scent. Diffusers come in a variety of styles, including ultrasonic, nebulizing, and heat-based models, and they may be utilized in homes, offices, or spas.

2. **Topical Applicability**: Diluted essential oils can be massaged into the skin or added to skincare products such as lotions, creams, and bath oils. To avoid skin sensitivity, essential oils should be diluted with a carrier oil (such as coconut, almond, or jojoba oil).

3. **Inhalation**: Adding a few drops of essential oil to a bowl of hot water or utilizing a personal inhaler can provide

Guide for somatic therapy

immediate relief for congestion, headaches, or stress.

4.**Sprays and Compresses**: Essential oils blended with water in a spray bottle or added to compresses can be used to refresh a space, create a tranquil environment, or for topical use in particular parts of the body.

Common Essential Oils and Their Applications*

Lavender: Lavender oil, known for its relaxing and soothing characteristics, is frequently used to relieve stress, induce relaxation, and enhance sleep quality.

Peppermint: Peppermint oil is invigorating and refreshing, and it can help relieve headaches, improve energy, and relieve nausea or muscular strain.

Guide for somatic therapy

Eucalyptus: Eucalyptus oil is often used to remove congestion, facilitate breathing, and enhance respiratory health due to its antibacterial characteristics.

Chamomile: Both Roman and German chamomile oils are prized for their relaxing properties, which aid in anxiety reduction, skin irritation relief, and relaxation.

Tea Tree: Tea tree oil is used for skin disorders, small wounds, acne, and as a natural home cleanser due to its antibacterial and antifungal qualities.

Benefits

Tension Reduction: Certain essential oils have relaxing properties that assist to relieve tension and anxiety while also promoting relaxation.

Guide for somatic therapy

Better Sleep: Lavender and other calming oils can help with sleep quality and insomnia alleviation.

Mood Enhancement: Aromas have the ability to impact emotions, boost moods, and promote a sense of well-being.

Pain Relief: Certain oils include analgesic characteristics that can help relieve headaches, muscular aches, and joint difficulties.

Considerations for Safety:
 Essential oils are very concentrated and should be used with caution. Always dilute them before application to the skin and test for allergies or skin problems with a patch test.
Pregnant women, young children, and those with specific medical problems should see a doctor before taking essential oils.

Guide for somatic therapy

Aromatherapy is a natural and enjoyable technique to improve one's well-being, whether for relaxation, mood enhancement, or a variety of health advantages. Exploring various essential oils and their uses may provide a wealth of olfactory pleasures as well as possible health benefits.

Journaling or Expressive Writing: Keeping a journal and writing down ideas, feelings, or concerns can help you express yourself and gain perspective. It promotes self-reflection and can be used as an emotional outlet.

Hobbies or pastimes that offer joy or relaxation, such as painting, gardening, listening to music, or physical activity such as yoga or walking, can be good self-soothing approaches.

Guide for somatic therapy

Relaxing sensory experiences:
Soothing sensory exercises engage your senses, promoting relaxation, stress reduction, and a relaxing influence on your mind and body. These activities center on sensory sensations that provide comfort and peace. Here's a more in-depth look at relaxing sensory activities:

1.**Warm baths or showers**:
A warm bath with bath salts, aromatic oils, or bubble bath can help to soothe muscles, relax the body, and relieve stress. Warm water showers can have a similar soothing effect.

2. **Listening to relaxing Music or Sounds**:
Listening to gentle, relaxing music, natural sounds, white noise, or instrumental melodies can help create a serene environment, decrease tension, and encourage relaxation.

Guide for somatic therapy

3. **Nature Engagement**: Spending time outside, whether in a park, garden, or simply sitting beneath a tree, may provide a sense of peace and connection with nature.

4. **Mindful Eating**: Taking the time to eat and appreciate food's flavors, textures, and scents may be a relaxing sensory experience. Concentrate on each mouthful, allowing it to fully activate your senses.

5. **Using Weighted Blankets**: Weighted blankets apply mild pressure on the body, providing relaxation and a sense of security. They can aid in the reduction of anxiety and the improvement of sleep quality.

6. **Drinking Herbal Tea**: A warm cup of herbal tea, such as chamomile or lavender, not only hydrates but also has relaxing properties and a pleasant scent.

Guide for somatic therapy

7. **Participating in Artistic or Creative Activities**:
Painting, painting, coloring, knitting, and other creative activities may be calming and a source of self-expression.

8. **Mindfulness Activities**: Mindfulness activities such as yoga, tai chi, or qigong involve slow movements, deep breathing, and focused attention, all of which promote relaxation and stress reduction.

9. **Using Sensory Tools**: Fidget toys, stress balls, or textured things such as worry stones or soft textiles can provide tactile sensations that help to relax the nervous system.

10.**Creating comfy Environments**: Surrounding oneself with soft blankets, comfy cushions, soothing colors, or dim lighting will help you create a nice and tranquil environment.

Guide for somatic therapy

Benefits of Relaxing Sensory Activities:

Stress Reduction: These activities induce relaxation, reduce stress hormones, and give a stress-relieving outlet.

Emotional Regulation: Using one's senses can help manage emotions and bring about a sense of peace in stressful times.

More Happiness:Regularly engaging in calming sensory activities can improve overall well-being by promoting a relaxed state of mind and body.

Incorporating these activities into your daily routine may help you generate moments of relaxation and serenity, providing a respite from the stresses of everyday life and creating a sense of peace and tranquility.

Guide for somatic therapy

Practices for Creating Stability.

Adopting habits that promote balance, resilience, and constancy in the face of life's changes and challenges is one way to achieve life stability. These activities promote emotional well-being, mental clarity, and a sense of security. Here's a comprehensive look at methods for establishing stability:

1. **Meditation and mindfulness:**
Daily Practice: Regularly practicing mindfulness or meditation improves mental clarity, decreases stress, and cultivates a sense of presence and tranquility.
Focused Attention: These techniques educate you to focus on the current moment, which promotes stability by anchoring your consciousness in the

Guide for somatic therapy

present rather than worrying about the past or future.

2. **Structure and routine:**

Regular pattern: Establishing a regular pattern can bring predictability and stability. Consistency in getting up, eating, working, and going to bed might help to develop a pleasant framework.

Prioritizing Tasks: Organizing tasks and assigning priority can aid in the management of obligations, decreasing stress and disarray.

3. **Practices for Physical Health:**

Regular Exercise: Physical activity, such as walking, yoga, or any other type of exercise, promotes stability by improving mood, lowering stress, and encouraging general well-being.

Healthy Eating: Nourishing your body with balanced meals supports physical health

Guide for somatic therapy

and provides sustained energy levels, which adds to stability.

4. **Emotional Control:**

Self-Reflection: Regular self-reflection aids in the understanding of emotions and reactions, improving emotional stability via self-awareness and resilience.

Coping methods: Learning good coping methods, such as deep breathing, journaling, or seeking assistance from loved ones, aids in the management of stress and emotional swings.

5. **Creating Support Networks:**

Connection: Developing relationships with supportive friends, family, or groups fosters a feeling of belonging and improves emotional stability via shared experiences and support.

Guide for somatic therapy

Professional Assistance: Seeking advice from therapists, counselors, or mentors can provide essential insights and strategies for dealing with issues and maintaining stability.

6. Setting Limits and Self-Care:

Healthy Boundaries: Having healthy boundaries in relationships and commitments promotes emotional stability by establishing a balance of personal needs and external obligations.

Self-Care Practices: Making self-care a priority, whether via relaxation, hobbies, or enjoyable activities, promotes mental and emotional well-being.

7.Lifelong Learning and Development:

Continuous Learning:Lifelong learning, whether through courses, books, or new experiences, promotes personal growth and

Guide for somatic therapy

flexibility, which contributes to stability through greater knowledge and skills.

8. **Gratitude and optimism:**

Practice thankfulness:Cultivating thankfulness by acknowledging and appreciating what you have helps stability by cultivating a positive mentality and resilience throughout difficult circumstances.

9. **Adaptability :**

Adaptability Skills: Developing the ability to adjust to change and be flexible in a variety of contexts improves stability by decreasing resistance to change and improving problem-solving abilities.

Stability is achieved by incorporating these activities throughout daily life, therefore providing a supporting framework that promotes emotional, bodily, and mental

Guide for somatic therapy

well-being. The combination of these behaviors promotes resilience, stability, and an overall sense of balance and happiness.

Keeping in touch with the present

Connecting to the present now is being totally involved and aware of what is going on right now, without being distracted by thoughts of the past or concerns about the future. Here's a thorough examination of strategies for connecting with the present moment:

1. **Meditation for Mindfulness:**
Focused Attention: Mindfulness meditation entails focusing on the breath, physiological

Guide for somatic therapy

sensations, or noises in order to bring your attention back to the present moment.
Observing Thoughts: Instead of becoming caught up in them, examine them objectively, allowing them to pass by like clouds in the sky.

2. **Mindfully Participating in Activities**:
Mindful Eating: Without distractions, pay full attention to the flavor, texture, and sensation of eating, savoring each mouthful.
3.Walking Meditation: Walk gently, paying attention to each step, the sensation of your feet on the ground, and your body movement.

4. **Awareness of one's own body and relaxation:**
Body Scan: Scrub your whole body from head to toe, noting regions of tension or relaxation and intentionally relaxing stiff muscles.

Guide for somatic therapy

Yoga or Tai Chi: These practices integrate movement, breath, and mindfulness, developing a stronger connection to the body and the present moment.

5. **Developing Gratitude:**

Gratitude Practice:Consider what you're grateful for, concentrating on the current gifts in your life rather than previous regrets or future concerns.

6. **Let Go of Your Judgment and Expectations:**

Non-Judgmental Observation: Practice watching your thoughts, feelings, and experiences without assigning them a positive or negative name.

Acceptance: Accept the current moment as it is, without attempting to alter it or wanting for it to be otherwise.

Guide for somatic therapy

7. **Acceptance and Mindfulness:**

Accepting Reality: Recognize that life unfolds in the present moment, and practice acceptance to find serenity in the midst of uncertainty.
Mindful Decision-Making: Make conscious choices and decisions by being completely present and taking into account the conditions of the moment.

8. **Participating Fully in Daily Activities:**

Pay Attention to Tasks: Whether it's work, housework, or pastimes, immerse yourself completely in what you're doing, paying attention to the intricacies and sensations involved.

9. **Distractions to Avoid:**
Reduce Multitasking: Do one activity at a time, limiting distractions to focus on the work at hand.

Guide for somatic therapy

10. **Reflective Practices**

Journaling: Writing down ideas, feelings, and experiences can aid in the processing of emotions and the awareness of the present moment.

Guide for somatic therapy

Guide for somatic therapy

Chapter 6

Breathing Exercises and Relaxation

Breathing and relaxation methods are effective strategies for stress reduction, mind-calming, and fostering a sense of relaxation and well-being. Here's a look at some different approaches:

1. **Exercises in Deep Breathing**

Diaphragmatic Breathing: Inhale deeply with your nose, causing your stomach to rise, then exhale slowly through your mouth, allowing your stomach to sink. Concentrate on taking deep, slow breaths.

4-7-8 Breathing:Inhale for four counts, hold for seven, and exhale for eight. Rep this

Guide for somatic therapy

pattern, enabling a soothing rhythm to settle your body and mind.

Box Breathing: Inhale, hold, exhale, and repeat for a total of four seconds. Make a square out of this design.

2. **PMR (Progressive Muscle Relaxation)**:

Tensing and Releasing Muscles:Tense and relax certain muscle groups for a few seconds. Move around your body systematically, releasing tension as you go to promote total relaxation.

4. **Meditation for Mindfulness:**

Focused Attention:Pay attention to your breath, sensations, or surroundings, allowing thoughts to pass through without judgment. This technique improves relaxation and relaxes the mind.

5. **Body Scan**

Muscle Scanning and Relaxation: Mentally scan your body from head to toe,

Guide for somatic therapy

detecting regions of tension. Then, intentionally relax each muscle group to relieve stress.

6. Autogenic Training
Self-Induced Relaxation: This approach promotes the body to relax by focusing on warmth, heaviness, and serenity in various body areas utilizing imagery and verbal cues.

7. Breath counting:
Counting Inhalations and Exhalations:Count each breath cycle, aiming for exhalations that are longer than inhalations. This technique promotes concentration and relaxation.

8. Yoga and Tai Chi:
Movement and Breath Integration:Gentle movement, breathing exercises, and mindfulness are used in these activities to promote relaxation and stress alleviation.

Guide for somatic therapy

9.**Aromatherapy Breathing:**
Inhaling Essential Oils: For further relaxation, combine deep breathing techniques with the use of relaxing essential fragrances such as lavender or chamomile.

10. **Stress Relieving Belly Breathing:**
Balanced Breathing: Put one hand on your chest and one on your stomach. Deeply inhale, feeling your abdomen rise and fall with each breath. This exercise induces the relaxation response.

Using these strategies on a daily basis will help you manage stress, reduce anxiety, and promote relaxation and peace. Experiment with several approaches to see which ones work best for you, and then include them into your regular routine to reap the most advantages.

Guide for somatic therapy

Somatic therapy applicable for peculiar cases

PTSD and Trauma

By incorporating the body's feelings and sensations into the healing process, somatic therapy provides a unique and successful way to resolving trauma and Post-Traumatic Stress Disorder (PTSD). Here's a more in-depth look at somatic therapy for trauma and PTSD:

Somatic Therapy in Trauma Healing:
Body-Centered Approach: Trauma is not only preserved in the mind, but also in body sensations, motions, and patterns, according to somatic therapy.

Resolving Physical Symptoms: It focuses on releasing and treating bodily symptoms of trauma, such as tightness,

Guide for somatic therapy

hypervigilance, or feeling estranged from one's body.

Somatic Therapy Techniques:
Somatic Experiencing (SE):SE was created by Peter Levine and focuses on recording physiological sensations and enabling the body to finish its normal self-regulating reactions to trauma.
Sensorimotor Psychotherapy: This method combines conversation therapy and body-based strategies to address how trauma affects body movements, sensations, and beliefs.

Addressing Fight-Flight-Freeze reactions:
Releasing Tension: Somatic therapy assists patients in releasing stored energy from fight-flight-freeze reactions by releasing muscle tension or permitting bodily movements associated with the initial trauma response.

Guide for somatic therapy

Neuroregulation: Techniques such as grounding, deep breathing, and gentle movement assist control the autonomic nervous system, minimizing hyperarousal or dissociation.

Increasing Body Awareness and Safety: Somatic therapy supports in reconnecting patients with body experiences, establishing a sense of safety, and increasing awareness of physical cues.

Resourcing and Self-Regulation:

Developing Internal Resources: Somatic therapy assists individuals in developing internal resources for self-soothing, resilience, and self-regulation during stressful situations.

Grounding Techniques: Clients are taught grounding activities to help them stay in the

Guide for somatic therapy

present moment and reduce overpowering sensations or memories.

Trauma Processing and Integration: Somatic Resourcing: Individuals acquire strategies to manage emotions and sensations before digging into traumatic memories, ensuring they feel secure and supported.

How to Integrate Traumatic Experiences:When clients feel more grounded and resilient, therapy may go forward to carefully explore and process painful memories or sensations, promoting integration and healing.

Long-Term Resilience and Healing: Encourage

Long-Term Well-Being:Somatic therapy attempts to promote overall well-being and

Guide for somatic therapy

increase an individual's resilience in dealing with future stresses, not simply symptoms.

Somatic therapy for trauma and PTSD stresses the body's critical role in healing by giving skills and strategies for processing trauma, regulating emotions, and restoring a sense of safety and connection with oneself. It is frequently useful when used in combination with other therapy modalities and administered by trauma-trained somatic therapists.

Anxiety and stress

Somatic therapy, which focuses on the feelings, movements, and experiences of the body, provides helpful solutions for reducing anxiety and stress. Here's an

Guide for somatic therapy

in-depth look at somatic therapy approaches for anxiety and stress management:

Body-Oriented Techniques:

Breathwork and Deep Relaxation: Deep breathing techniques, such as diaphragmatic breathing or 4-7-8 breathing, soothe the nervous system and reduce anxiety and tension.

PMR (Progressive Muscle Relaxation): This method includes systematically tensing and releasing muscle regions, encouraging physical relaxation and relieving stress.

Grounding and Mindfulness Practices:

Sensory Grounding: Focusing on sights, sounds, touch, taste, or smell to anchor

Guide for somatic therapy

oneself in the present moment, lessening feelings of detachment and anxiety.

Mindful Awareness: Techniques such as body scans and mindfulness meditation encourage present-moment awareness, which reduces rumination and unpleasant thoughts.

Movement-Based Therapies:
Yoga and Tai Chi: These practices integrate movement, breathwork, and mindfulness to promote relaxation, reduce muscular tension, and soothe the mind.

Dance Therapy or Expressive Movement: Encourages unrestricted movement and expression, allowing stored tension and emotions to be released and stress levels to be reduced.

Somatic Experiencing (SE): SE focuses on detecting and releasing bodily feelings

Guide for somatic therapy

linked with anxiety, allowing the body to finish interrupted fight-or-flight reactions and restore balance.

Body-Centered Stress Reduction: Trauma-Informed Approaches: Addressing stress and anxiety with body-based strategies that take into account previous traumatic experiences and their influence on the body's stress response.

Body Awareness Training: Fostering proactive stress management by increasing awareness of physical sensations, movements, and stress indicators.

Regulation of the Autonomic Nervous System:
Polyvagal Theory Applications: Using polyvagal theory-aligned approaches to

Guide for somatic therapy

control the autonomic nervous system, encouraging relaxation and lowering the body's stress reaction.

Self-Soothing and Resourcing:

Building Internal Resources:Learning self-soothing methods, creating safe internal spaces, and developing resilience to manage stress and anxiety triggers are all examples of building internal resources.

Anchoring in the Present: Using grounding techniques to anchor oneself in the present moment, minimizing anxiety about future or previous occurrences.

Integrating the Body-Mind Connection:

Recognizing and treating the interdependence of physiological sensations and emotional experiences, encouraging balance and minimizing anxiety symptoms.

Guide for somatic therapy

Developing a Self-Care Routine

Developing a self-care regimen might appear to be a difficult job, especially when suffering with worry and stress.

But you're making time to look after the most important person in your life: yourself.

Even five minutes a day may make a significant impact in terms of long-term improvement and putting yourself in command of your mental health and well-being. It also assists you in re establishing contact with your inner child, who is frequently neglected and pushed aside while we are preoccupied with our everyday activities.

Here are some excellent suggestions:

- Take a break from social media and digital gadgets.
- Get a book and read it.

Guide for somatic therapy

- Spend some time in nature.
- After work, treat yourself to a relaxing bubble bath.
- For a relaxing ambiance, use some candles or incense.

Depression

By incorporating the body's feelings, sensations, and movements into the therapeutic process, somatic therapy provides important techniques to address depression. Here's a thorough examination of somatic therapy approaches for depression management:

1. **Body-Mind Integration**:

Guide for somatic therapy

Understanding the Body-Mind Connection: Recognizing the link between physiological sensations and emotional states, and investigating how physical experiences influence mood and vice versa.

2. **Breathwork and Relaxation Techniques**: Diaphragmatic breathing, box breathing, or 4-7-8 breathing soothe the nervous system, lower stress hormones, and improve depression symptoms.
Progressive Muscle Relaxation (PMR): Tensing and relaxing muscle groups promotes physical relaxation, alleviating physical tension linked with sadness.

Releasing Stored Tension: Somatic experiencing approaches are designed to identify and release bodily feelings associated with prior traumatic or painful events that contribute to depressive symptoms.

Guide for somatic therapy

Movement-Based Therapies:

Yoga, Tai Chi, or Qigong: Using movement, breath, and mindfulness to relax, reduce muscular tension, and boost mood by releasing endorphins.

Dance or Movement Therapy:Promotes expressive movement, emotional release, and general well-being.

Mindfulness and Grounding Practices:

Sensory Grounding: Using one's senses to anchor oneself in the present moment, minimizing depressed rumination and developing a feeling of presence.

Mindfulness Meditation: Concentrating on present-moment awareness aids in the management of depressed thoughts and promotes the acceptance of feelings without judgment.

Guide for somatic therapy

Body-Centered Stress Reduction:

Stress Reduction Techniques:Addressing stress-related symptoms through body-based treatments, therefore assisting in the reduction of overall discomfort, which contributes to depression.

Self-Soothing and Resourcing:

Developing Self-Soothing Techniques:Developing self-compassion practices, inner resource building, and resilience to handle depression symptoms.

Creating Safe Internal Spaces:Developing techniques to manage emotions during depressed periods and cultivating a sense of safety and comfort inside oneself.

Guide for somatic therapy

Trauma-Informed Approaches: Exploring prior Trauma Impact: Investigating how prior traumatic experiences stored in the body may contribute to depressive symptoms, with the goal of releasing stored trauma.

Body Awareness and Self-Care: Developing awareness of bodily sensations, fostering self-care activities, and recognizing physical requirements to promote mental health are all examples of increasing body awareness.

Enhancing Emotional Regulation: Techniques for identifying and regulating emotions by focusing on physical sensations, boosting emotional self-regulation.

Somatic therapy for depression strives to incorporate body-centered techniques into established therapeutic procedures,

Guide for somatic therapy

encouraging healing and building a holistic knowledge of depression. These activities enable people to develop more self-awareness, control emotions, relieve tension, and build resilience in order to successfully manage depressive symptoms. Seeking the help of a trained somatic therapist can give individualized therapies to address individual needs while also promoting general well-being.

Emotional control

Somatic exercises serve an important role in emotional regulation by integrating body sensations with emotions, assisting individuals in identifying, understanding, and effectively managing their feelings. Here are

Guide for somatic therapy

some somatic exercises that might help you regulate your emotions:

Body Scanning:

Procedure:
Lie down or sit in a comfortable position. Scanning your body from head to toe, take note of any places of tension, discomfort, or relaxation.

Benefits:
Body scanning raises awareness of body sensations associated with emotions, allowing you to detect regions of tension or serenity and make appropriate modifications.

Grounding Techniques:

Process:
To anchor oneself to the present now, use grounding techniques such as focused

Guide for somatic therapy

breathing, pushing your feet firmly into the ground, or holding onto an item.

Benefits:
Grounding techniques assist in shifting focus away from overpowering emotions and into the current surroundings, lowering anxiety and increasing emotional stability.

Breathwork:
Process: Engage in deep breathing exercises such as diaphragmatic breathing or box breathing, emphasizing slow, deep inhales and exhales.

Benefits: Controlled breathing calms emotions, reduces tension, and promotes relaxation by regulating the neurological system.

Somatic Experiencing (SE):

Process: SE procedures entail recording physiological experiences associated with certain emotions. Individuals perceive bodily

Guide for somatic therapy

reactions associated with emotions without passing judgment.

Benefits: SE assists with the processing and regulation of emotions by monitoring and acknowledging body sensations, hence lowering the intensity of emotional reactions.

Movement and Expression:

Process: Engage in expressive movement activities such as dance, yoga, or tai chi to express emotions via physical movements.
Benefits: Movement-based activities enhance a sense of well-being and emotional balance by releasing accumulated tension and facilitating emotional discharge.

Progressive Muscle Relaxation (PMR):

Guide for somatic therapy

Process: Tense and release different muscle groups methodically, beginning with the toes and working your way up to the head, observing feelings in each muscle group.

Benefits: PMR alleviates muscular tension associated with stress and anxiety, improving relaxation and assisting with emotional control.

Self-Soothing contact:

Process: To offer reassurance and comfort, use mild self-massage methods or soothing contact, such as embracing oneself or resting a palm over the heart.

Benefits: Self-soothing touch triggers the relaxation response in the body, creating feelings of safety and calm during emotional discomfort.

Body-Based Visualization:

Guide for somatic therapy

Process: Imagine a safe, relaxing setting or visualize physically releasing emotions, enabling the body to react in a supportive atmosphere.

Benefits: Visualization methods involve both the mind and the body, enabling emotional control and anxiety reduction.

These somatic exercises promote a stronger link between the body and emotions, providing useful tools for identifying, regulating, and controlling emotions. Regular practice increases self-awareness, enables individuals to respond to emotions adaptively, and promotes general emotional well-being. Consultation with a somatic therapist or other qualified expert can give specific exercises to meet individual requirements and assist with emotional control.

Guide for somatic therapy

Eating Disorders and Body Image:

Somatic therapy, which focuses on the mind-body connection and how it pertains to one's relationship with their body, is a beneficial strategy for resolving body image problems and eating disorders. Here's a detailed look at somatic treatment approaches for various issues:

Body Awareness and Mindfulness:

Sensory Exploration: Somatic treatment encourages people to explore their bodies' experiences without judgment, which leads to increased body awareness and mindfulness.

Mindful Eating: Mindfulness practice while eating assists individuals in connecting with biological cues of hunger and satiety, establishing a healthy connection with food.

Guide for somatic therapy

Grounding Exercises: Grounding practices, such as deep breathing or connecting with the current moment, help people anchor themselves in the present moment, lowering concern over body image.

Somatic Experiencing (SE):

Tracking Bodily Sensations: SE entails investigating bodily sensations associated with emotions and body image, assisting in the processing of underlying trauma or emotional distress that contributes to disordered eating.
Releasing Tension:SE techniques aid in the release of accumulated tension and stress reactions related to poor body image views.

Embodied Movement and Expression:

Guide for somatic therapy

Yoga or Dance Therapy:Movement-based activities encourage positive body acceptance, self-expression, and connection with the body.

Expressive Arts:Using creative forms of expression, such as art therapy or body mapping, allows people to explore their views and emotions about their bodies in a safe environment.

Self-Compassion and Acceptance:

Cultivating Self-Compassion:Somatic therapy teaches people to be kind and accepting of themselves and their bodies.

Creating a Positive Body Narrative: Shifting attention away from negative body ideas and toward identifying and enjoying the body's strengths and possibilities.

Guide for somatic therapy

Trauma-Informed Approaches:

Addressing Underlying Trauma:Somatic therapy investigates prior traumas or adversities that contribute to distorted body image or disordered eating practices.

Healing Through the Body:Techniques for releasing buried trauma from the body encourage healing and assist in the resolution of linked body image and eating issues.

 Body-Centered Self-Care:
Gentle Body Work: Practicing gentle self-massage or body-centered relaxation methods promotes self-care and body nourishment.

Mind-Body Connection: Somatic therapy aids in the integration of the mind and body, establishing a healthy relationship and

Guide for somatic therapy

narrowing the gap between ideas and physiological experiences.

Somatic therapy is a comprehensive approach that takes into account the interaction of ideas, emotions, and physical experiences in relation to body image and eating disorders. By addressing the underlying emotional and physical factors that contribute to these issues, these strategies attempt to build self-awareness, promote self-acceptance, and enable healing. Working with a qualified somatic therapist or mental health practitioner who specializes in these areas can provide persons trying to better their relationship with their bodies and eating patterns with individualized therapies and support.

Relationship difficulties: By concentrating on the mind-body link and how it affects relational dynamics, somatic therapy provides useful tools and ways for

Guide for somatic therapy

addressing relationship difficulties. Here's an in-depth look at somatic therapy approaches for relationship improvement:

Recognizing Nonverbal Cues: Somatic therapy focuses on nonverbal communication, assisting patients in recognizing and interpreting their own and others' body language and gestures.

Increasing Body Awareness: Techniques are designed to increase awareness of body sensations, assisting in the recognition of emotional reactions and promoting sympathetic understanding in relationships.

Emotion Regulation and Co-Regulation: Somatic exercises teach people how to manage their emotions by observing their physical sensations and practicing skills such as breathwork and grounding.

Guide for somatic therapy

Relationship Co-Regulation: Learning to manage one's own emotions can improve interactions and develop stronger emotional co-regulation within partnerships.

Attachment and Relational Patterns:
Exploring Attachment Styles: Somatic therapy investigates how early attachment experiences impact contemporary relational patterns, assisting individuals in understanding and dealing with attachment-related issues.

Reprocessing Trauma in Relationships:Somatic Experiencing techniques help in the processing of relational trauma held in the body, which contributes to relationship issues.

Body-Centered Couples or Family Therapy:Couples or families may participate in somatic therapy sessions, which focus on body-centered strategies to

Guide for somatic therapy

treat marital difficulties or communication challenges.

Facilitating Connection: Couples or family members participate in connection-building exercises such as synchronized breathing or mirroring motions, which enhance understanding and empathy.

Boundary Setting and Empowerment:

Healthy limits:Somatic therapy may help people recognize and set healthy limits in their relationships, encouraging mutual respect and emotional safety.

Empowerment Techniques:Techniques that assist individuals in asserting their wants and preferences, promoting a sense of empowerment in relationships.

Resourcing and Strengthening Connection:

Guide for somatic therapy

Building Resources: Somatic exercises assist couples and individuals in developing internal resources for dealing with relationship difficulties and creating resilience.

Improving Connection: Touch, eye contact, and nonverbal gestures are used to improve connection, boosting closeness and understanding.

Trauma-Informed Relationship Therapy: Addressing Relational Trauma: Somatic therapy investigates how previous relational traumas affect contemporary relationships, assisting in the resolution of unresolved issues and the improvement of relational dynamics.

Somatic therapy takes a unique approach to relationship improvement by recognizing the interdependence of the mind and body within relational dynamics. These strategies

Guide for somatic therapy

try to improve communication, increase empathy, encourage emotional control, and address underlying issues that contribute to relationship difficulties. Seeking help from a certified somatic therapist or relationship counselor can provide tailored solutions to address specific relational challenges and build better, more rewarding relationships.

Self-esteem and self-assurance

Somatic therapy focuses on the mind-body link and how it impacts one's self-perception to give effective ways for increasing self-esteem and self-confidence. Here's a more in-depth look at the impact of somatic therapy in enhancing self-esteem and self-confidence:

Guide for somatic therapy

Body Awareness and Acceptance:
Enhancing Body Awareness: Somatic therapy promotes acceptance of oneself without judgment or criticism by encouraging awareness of body sensations and emotions.

Embracing the Body: Techniques encourage people to appreciate their bodies' strengths and capacities, moving the emphasis away from perceived imperfections and toward self-acceptance.

Empowerment Through Movement:
Embodied Empowerment: Participating in movement-based activities such as yoga or dance therapy may help people feel empowered and in control of their body.
Confidence in Movement: Promoting confident body language and posture promotes self-confidence and a positive self-image.

Guide for somatic therapy

Trauma-Informed Approaches:
Addressing Underlying Trauma: Somatic therapy investigates how prior traumas or negative experiences affect self-esteem, assisting clients in processing and releasing stored trauma from the body.

Building Resilience: Techniques focus on developing resilience and inner strength, allowing people to overcome negative self-perceptions based on prior experiences.

Self-Compassion and Self-Care:
Self-Compassion Cultivation: Somatic therapy enables people to cultivate self-compassion, cultivating kindness and understanding for themselves.
Self-Care Promotion: Self-soothing methods such as self-massage or relaxation exercises, as well as fostering self-care and nourishing the self, are examples of techniques.

Guide for somatic therapy

Confidence-Building exercises:Skill Development:Somatic treatment includes exercises targeted at improving skills, talents, and capacities, as well as raising confidence through mastery and success.

Good Reinforcement: Highlighting and appreciating personal victories and achievements promotes self-esteem and a good self-image.

Empowering Assertiveness and limits: Assertiveness Training: Techniques assist individuals in developing assertiveness skills, allowing them to boldly state demands and limits in relationships.

Boundary Setting: Learning to create and maintain healthy boundaries promotes self-esteem and empowerment.

Body-Centered Self-Expression: Expressive Arts Therapy: Using artistic

Guide for somatic therapy

expressions to communicate and process emotions promotes self-expression and self-discovery.

Voice and Motion:Techniques such as vocal exercises and movement activities promote self-expression, allowing people to discover and affirm their voice and individuality.

Mind-Body Integration:

Mind-Body Harmonization:Somatic therapy seeks to integrate ideas, emotions, and physical experiences in order to promote a balanced and aligned sense of self.

Somatic therapy promotes a comprehensive approach that recognizes the inextricable link between the mind and body in the development of self-esteem and self-confidence. These approaches build a good self-image and a higher sense of

Guide for somatic therapy

confidence and value by encouraging self-awareness, self-acceptance, resilience, and empowerment. Seeking the help of a professional somatic therapist can provide individualized therapies to address specific self-esteem and self-confidence difficulties while also promoting general personal growth and well-being.

Loss and grief

Somatic therapy helps people cope with sorrow and loss by identifying and resolving the physical and emotional effects of these events on the body. Here's a more in-depth look at how somatic therapy might help with sorrow and loss:

Embodied Grieving:
Acknowledging Bodily Sensations: Somatic therapy helps people to identify and

Guide for somatic therapy

explore bodily symptoms of grieving, such as heaviness, tightness, or numbness.

Honoring Emotional Responses:

Techniques aid in understanding and embracing emotional responses stored in the body, enabling validation and normality of mourning emotions.

Body-Centered Awareness:

Breathwork and Relaxation:During times of mourning, deep breathing exercises and progressive muscle relaxation methods can help reduce physical tension and promote calm.

Mindful Presence: Practicing mindfulness and grounding activities can help you stay present and manage l
overwhelming grief-related emotions.

Somatic Experiencing (SE) for Grief:

Releasing held Trauma:SE techniques aid in the release of trauma associated with loss

Guide for somatic therapy

held in the body, allowing for the processing and integration of painful emotions.

Completing Unfinished Responses:Facilitating the completion of interrupted or suppressed emotional responses linked with the loss.

Expressive Movement and Creativity:
Movement as Expression: Taking part in movement therapies or expressive arts helps people to express and process their feelings nonverbally, which promotes release and healing.
Creative Expression:Activities such as art therapy or journaling allow for emotional expression and investigation, which can help with the mourning process.

Trauma-Informed grieving Support:
Addressing prior Trauma:Somatic therapy investigates how prior traumas may enhance grieving reactions, assisting

Guide for somatic therapy

individuals in addressing unresolved trauma associated with the loss.

Healing Through the Body: Techniques that focus on releasing accumulated sorrow and trauma from the body in order to promote healing and acceptance.

Self-Care and Nurturing Practices:

Self-Soothing Techniques: Encouragement of gentle self-massage, relaxation exercises, or participation in activities that give comfort and nurture throughout the mourning process.

Supporting Resilience: Developing coping techniques for managing grief triggers and building resources to support resilience.

Body-Mind Integration and Meaning-Making:

Holistic Integration: Somatic therapy combines thoughts, emotions, and bodily sensations, allowing for a more

Guide for somatic therapy

comprehensive knowledge of grief and its effects on the individual.

Finding Meaning: Techniques assist individuals in discovering personal meaning and incorporating loss into their life story, encouraging a feeling of closure and continuity.

Grief Group Somatic Therapy:

Shared Expression: Individuals can discuss and process their grieving experiences in group sessions, giving mutual support and a sense of belonging.

Somatic therapy acknowledges the importance of the mind-body link in the mourning process and provides a compassionate and comprehensive approach to sorrow and loss. These strategies attempt to help people navigate sorrow by encouraging self-awareness, acceptance, and healing, as well as finding meaningful ways to acknowledge and

Guide for somatic therapy

incorporate loss into their life. Seeking the help of a competent somatic therapist or grief counselor can provide individualized therapies to meet unique needs and support healing throughout the mourning process.

Adaptability and coping abilities

Somatic therapy focuses on enhancing an individual's ability to adapt, recover from stresses, and thrive in tough conditions by integrating the mind and body. Here's an in-depth look at somatic therapy practices designed to promote resilience and coping:

Breathwork and Relaxation Techniques:
Using deep breathing exercises, diaphragmatic breathing, or progressive muscle relaxation helps regulate the nervous system, lowering tension and encouraging calm.

Guide for somatic therapy

Grounding Practices:Techniques such as grounding exercises and mindfulness help to anchor people to the present moment, giving stability during times of stress or worry.

Self-Soothing and Emotional Regulation:
Sensory Awareness: Somatic therapy raises awareness of physical sensations associated with emotions, allowing for early identification of stress responses and increasing self-regulation.
Self-Care Techniques: Self-care methods such as mild self-massage, soothing touch, or relaxation exercises help to manage stress and promote emotional well-being.

Trauma-Informed Approaches:
Addressing Past Trauma:Techniques try to detect and release stored trauma from the

Guide for somatic therapy

body, therefore minimizing the influence of previous events on present stress reactions.

Developing Resilience: Somatic therapy helps people build inner resources and strength, which helps them cope with pressures and problems.

Embodied Empowerment:

Embodied Practices: Movement-based treatments such as yoga, tai chi, or dance encourage a sense of empowerment and mastery over the body, boosting confidence and resilience.

Assertiveness and Boundaries:Techniques assist individuals in asserting boundaries and boldly expressing demands, resulting in a better sense of control and resilience in relationships.

Guide for somatic therapy

Mind-Body Integration and Coping Strategies:

Holistic Integration:Somatic therapy combines thoughts, emotions, and physical sensations, promoting a more balanced understanding and reaction to stresses.

Development of Coping methods: Encouraging the development of coping methods that are matched with physiological experiences, allowing for adaptive reactions to stresses.

Resourcing and Strengthening:

Building Internal Resources: Practices focus on cultivating one's own strengths, good characteristics, and resilience elements, fostering a sense of personal empowerment.

Guide for somatic therapy

Support Systems and Social Connection: Techniques assist in identifying and utilizing support networks, developing resilience via social connection and community.

Growth mentality and Meaning-Making:
Promoting progress: Somatic treatment fosters a growth mentality, allowing people to see problems as opportunities for learning and progress.
Determining Meaning: Techniques assist individuals in finding meaning and purpose in adversity, which contributes to resilience and emotional strength.

By incorporating body-centered practices into daily life, somatic therapy enables patients to develop resilience and coping abilities. These techniques develop resilience and general well-being by encouraging self-awareness, emotional control, empowerment, and adaptive reactions to stresses. Seeking the help of a

Guide for somatic therapy

professional somatic therapist can give individualized therapies to help develop coping strategies and resilience in the face of life's obstacles.

Using somatic treatment in conjunction with other techniques

When somatic therapy is combined with other modalities, a comprehensive and holistic approach to addressing all areas of an individual's well-being is created. This combination enables a more nuanced and tailored treatment strategy that capitalizes on the benefits of several therapeutic techniques. Here's an investigation on combining somatic treatment with several modalities:

Guide for somatic therapy

1. **Cognitive Behavioral Therapy (CBT) and Somatic Therapy**:

Addressing Thoughts and Bodily Sensations: Combining CBT's cognitive restructuring with somatic techniques allows people to challenge negative thoughts while also addressing associated bodily sensations for a more comprehensive approach to healing.

Changes in Behavior and Bodily Reactions: Integrating CBT behavioral therapies with somatic awareness assists in the modification of behaviors associated with physiological suffering, enabling holistic transformation.

2.**Mindfulness and Somatic Therapy**:Incorporating mindfulness techniques into somatic treatment improves body-centered awareness, encouraging

Guide for somatic therapy

increased awareness of physical sensations and emotions.

Meditation for Somatic Mindfulness: Using somatic awareness techniques in conjunction with mindfulness meditation fosters a stronger link between body experiences and present-moment consciousness.

3. **Expressive Arts treatments with Somatic Techniques:**
Creative Expression and Somatic Awareness: By combining somatic practices with expressive arts treatments such as painting or dance therapy, nonverbal investigation and expression of physical feelings and emotions is possible.

Combining Movement and Creativity:Using movement-based expressive arts activities in conjunction with

Guide for somatic therapy

somatic therapy promotes a deeper investigation of emotions held in the body.

4. Psychodynamic treatment with Somatic Approaches:
Exploring Past Experiences: Combining somatic approaches with psychodynamic treatment assists in the exploration and processing of emotions and memories held in the body from previous experiences.

Understanding Unconscious Patterns: Addressing unconscious patterns and defenses via psychodynamic inquiry and somatic awareness contributes to a more holistic therapy approach.

5. **Trauma-Informed Approaches and Somatic Therapy:**
Trauma Resolution and Somatic Healing: Combining trauma-informed treatments, such as EMDR or Sensorimotor Psychotherapy, with somatic approaches

Guide for somatic therapy

aids in the resolution of trauma stored in the body.

Comprehensive Trauma Healing: Combining trauma-focused techniques with somatic therapy promotes a comprehensive approach to emotional and physical trauma rehabilitation.

6. **Bodywork and Somatic Experiences: Massage treatment and Somatic Techniques**: During treatment sessions, combining massage or bodywork with somatic therapy promotes relaxation, reduces physical tension, and increases body-centered awareness.

Acupuncture or Acupressure as a Somatic Practice Complement: Acupuncture or acupressure used in conjunction with somatic treatments helps to regulate energy flow and aids in stress reduction and emotional management.

Guide for somatic therapy

7. **Integrative Self-Care Approaches:**
Self-Compassion Practices: Combining somatic therapy with self-compassion practices improves self-care and cultivates a loving and welcoming attitude toward body experiences and emotions.

Holistic Self-Regulation: Combining somatic activities with self-regulation approaches such as breathwork or mindfulness aids in holistic emotional regulation and stress management.

When somatic therapy is combined with other modalities, a synergistic approach is created that addresses the complex aspect of an individual's experiences. This integration recognizes the mind-body link, allowing for a more thorough understanding and treatment of emotional, psychological, and physical well-being. Collaboration among skilled specialists in various modalities provides individualized and personalized treatments, assisting

Guide for somatic therapy

individuals on their path to holistic healing
and progress.

Chapter 7

Developing Your Own Somatic Self-Care Plan

Creating a tailored routine that focuses on nurturing and attention to your body's needs, sensations, and overall well-being is the first step in developing a somatic self-care strategy. Here's a comprehensive guide on creating a somatic self-care plan:

1. **Assess Your Needs and Goals:**
Self-Reflection: Consider your present stresses, emotional triggers, and bodily sensations associated with stress or discomfort.
Set Goals: Decide what you want to accomplish with your self-care strategy,

Guide for somatic therapy

whether it's stress reduction, emotional regulation, or increased general well-being.

2. **Body Awareness and Somatic techniques**: Experiment with various somatic techniques such as deep breathing, progressive muscle relaxation, and body scan meditation.
Notice Bodily Sensations:Become aware of how your body reacts to stress and relaxation, identifying regions of tension and ease.

3. **Create a Routine:**
Consistency is Essential: Make time for self-care techniques on a regular basis, including them into your daily or weekly routine.

Construct Rituals: Make self-care activities a natural and joyful part of your day by creating rituals around them.

Guide for somatic therapy

4. **Mindfulness and Grounding Techniques:**

Mindful Moments: To anchor yourself in the present now, include mindfulness activities throughout your day, whether at meals, while walking, or during breaks.

Grounding Exercises: To center oneself during times of stress or overwhelm, use grounding techniques such as deep breathing or sensory stimuli.

5.**Movement and Body-Centered Activities:**

Select Movement Practices: To increase body awareness and relaxation, engage in movement-based activities that connect with you, such as yoga, dancing, or tai chi.

Mindful Exercise:

Instead of pushing for results, practice exercises deliberately, paying attention to sensations and breathing.

6. **Self-Care Strategies:**

Guide for somatic therapy

Gentle Self-Massage: Apply gentle self-massage methods to particular parts of the body to relieve tension and promote relaxation and comfort.

Soothing Activities: To encourage relaxation, incorporate soothing sensory experiences such as aromatherapy, warm baths, or listening to quiet music.

7. Boundaries and Self-Compassion:

Set Boundaries: Set boundaries to safeguard your physical and emotional well-being, as well as recognize when to say no and prioritize your needs.

Experience Self-Compassion: When executing your self-care strategy, be kind with yourself, allowing for flexibility and self-forgiveness.

8. Comprehensive Approach and Support Systems Whole-Person Approach: In your self-care plan, address physical, emotional,

Guide for somatic therapy

mental, and spiritual needs to ensure a comprehensive approach to well-being.

Seek Support: When required, reach out to helpful friends, family, or experts, understanding the need of external support in self-care.

9.Regular Evaluation and Adjustment:

Assess and Adapt:Assess and adapt your self-care routines on a regular basis, tweaking or modifying activities as needed to better suit your changing requirements.

Experiment and Explore: Be open to experimenting with new somatic techniques or approaches, allowing for discovery and growth in your self-care journey.

10.Self-Reflection and Gratitude:

Reflect on Progress: Take time to reflect on how your self-care strategy is affecting your well-being, recognizing good

Guide for somatic therapy

developments as well as places for additional improvement.

Practice Gratitude:Develop gratitude for the work you make to care for yourself, acknowledging and appreciating your dedication to self-care.

A dedication to fostering your body-mind connection and prioritizing your well-being is required when developing a somatic self-care strategy. Customize your plan to meet your own needs and interests, and allow it to change as you continue on your path to holistic self-care and well-being. Remember that self-compassion and patience are vital during this process.

Guide for somatic therapy

The need for safety and boundaries

In somatic therapy, safety and limits serve as the foundation for a stable and comfortable environment in which to explore your emotional and bodily experiences. Here's why they're so crucial:

1.**A sense of safety and comfort**: Consider entering into a comfortable area where you feel completely protected and relaxed. That's the feeling we strive for in somatic therapy, so you may feel at ease and open up.

2. **Believing in Your Therapist**: It's like having a good buddy you can rely on. Building a trusting connection with your therapist is vital for feeling secure to

express and explore your innermost feelings.

3. **Your Comfort Zone Is Important**: Consider it like respecting your personal bubble! During the sessions, you get to select what feels right and what doesn't. Your therapist is attentive and considerate of your feelings and boundaries.

4. **Gently Handling Tough Stuff**: We sometimes need to talk about unpleasant topics. Safety and limits assist ensure that we go at a speed that feels comfortable for you and does not become too overwhelming.

5. **A sense of empowerment and control**: It's like taking the wheel of your own car. You're in control with safety and boundaries. You select how much or how little you want to explore, and your therapist will guide you through the process.

Guide for somatic therapy

6. **Ensuring Your Safety**: Your therapist, like a good friend who checks in on you, is concerned about how you're feeling. They are there to assist you feel better and more at ease if anything doesn't feel right.

7.**Maintaining Respect and Professionalism**: Your therapist is also aware of the limits. They ensure that everything remains professional and focused on making you feel better. It's all about establishing a secure and comfortable environment particularly for you.

In a word, safety and limits in somatic therapy are similar to having a comfortable and secure environment where you can be yourself and focus on feeling better without feeling pressured. It's all about you feeling secure, appreciated, and in control of your healing and feeling good journey.

Guide for somatic therapy

Guide for somatic therapy

Chapter 8

Other somatic exercise

1.**Body scan meditation**: is a mindfulness technique that includes bringing attention to different regions of the body in a methodical manner, recognizing sensations, and fostering calm. Here's a more in-depth look into body scan meditation:

Setting the Scene:

Comfortable Position: Locate a comfortable position, lying down or sitting, where you may rest without being distracted.

Mindful Awareness: Begin by becoming aware of your breath and allowing yourself to relax and quiet down.

Beginning the Body Scan

Systematic Focus:Begin at one end of your body, either the toes or the crown of your head, and gradually transfer your focus through each body component.

Attention and Observation: Pay close attention to each place, noting any feelings without judgment. it might be warmth, tension, tingling, or even a lack of sensation.

Gentle Attention:

Guided Visualization: Some methods include guided audio or vocal cues to assist in directing attention through the body, so fostering relaxation and awareness.

Relaxation and Release:Intentionally relax and release any tension in each body area, allowing it to soften and let go.

Non judgemental Observation

Sensation Acceptance: Practice accepting whatever sensations emerge without

Guide for somatic therapy

classifying them as pleasant or harmful. The goal is just to observe what is present.

Remaining Present: If your mind wanders or ideas occur, gently bring your attention back to the sensations in the current body location.

Developing Body Awareness:

Increased Sensory Awareness: Body scan meditation fosters a stronger connection between mind and body by increasing awareness of physical sensations.

Reducing Tension: The practice improves bodily relaxation and a sense of general tranquility by actively easing regions of tension.

Finishing the Practice:

Gradual Return: After scanning your complete body, take a few seconds to sense your body as a whole and your connection to the surface that is supporting you.

Guide for somatic therapy

Slow Re-entry: If your eyes are closed, slowly open them and gradually bring your consciousness back to the current moment.

Body scan meditation is an excellent technique for stress reduction, relaxation, and cultivating a greater awareness of the body's feelings. It facilitates the identification of regions of tension, allowing for purposeful relaxation and release, which can contribute to an overall sense of well-being. Body scan meditation, when practiced consistently, can help people establish a deeper mind-body connection and a more tranquil relationship with their bodily experiences.

2. **Feldenkrais Technique**:
The Feldenkrais Method is an educational technique established by Dr. Moshe Feldenkrais that focuses on movement, bodily awareness, and self-improvement. It attempts to promote general well-being by increasing self-awareness and improving

Guide for somatic therapy

movement ability. Here's a more in-depth look at the Feldenkrais Method:

Awareness Through Movement(ATM) refers to the ability to be aware of yourself.

Soft Movements: The approach employs slow, soft movements and sequences that explore various movement patterns, improving flexibility, coordination, and posture.

Mindful Exploration: Individuals are encouraged to pay close attention to their movements, sensations, and interactions with the environment through guided verbal instructions.

Functional Integration (FI):

private Sessions: In FI, a professional practitioner tailors movements and addresses unique requirements or limits of the client through gentle touch and vocal coaching.

Guide for somatic therapy

Personalized Approach: The practitioner's primary focus is on refining movement patterns, increasing body awareness, and promoting simpler, more efficient methods of moving.

Feldenkrais Principles:

Brain Plasticity: The ability of the brain to adapt and rearrange movement patterns via awareness and careful investigation is emphasized.

Effortless Movement: Encourages movement in the most efficient and least effortful way possible, avoiding unneeded tension and strain.

Mind-Body Connection

Increased Sensory Awareness: The approach encourages heightened sensory experience, which leads to a better knowledge of how movements feel and how they affect the body.

Guide for somatic therapy

Mindful Movement Practices: By being more aware of habitual motions, people may experiment with new, more comfortable ways to move, lowering stress on the body.

Benefits of Feldenkrais :

Improved Movement Quality: Improves flexibility, coordination, and balance by resolving movement constraints and increasing overall movement ease.
Pain Reduction: Promotes more efficient and pleasant movement patterns, which aids in the reduction of pain associated with chronic diseases or accidents.
Enhanced Well-Being:Increased bodily awareness promotes relaxation, decreases tension, and creates a sense of general well-being.

Application in a Variety of Situations
Performance Enhancement: Athletes, musicians, and performers use performance
Guide for somatic therapy

enhancement to fine-tune movement abilities, prevent injuries, and increase performance.

Rehabilitation: Used in rehabilitation settings to promote gentle movement and improve body awareness in order to facilitate recovery from injuries or procedures.

The Feldenkrais Method is a gentle yet effective method for enhancing mobility, developing body awareness, and boosting general well-being. Individuals can find new, more comfortable ways of moving, decreasing strain and improving their quality of life via mindful movement exploration. The practice stresses the significance of self-awareness, ease of movement, and the mind-body link in achieving enhanced physical and mental well-being, whether used for rehabilitation, performance enhancement, or just personal growth.

Guide for somatic therapy

3. **Alexander Technique (AT):**

This is a way of re-educating the body to move more effectively and smoothly, with the goal of increasing movement coordination, posture, and general well-being. Invented by F.M. It stresses mindfulness, self-awareness, and intentional control over movement patterns, as taught by Alexander. Here's a more in-depth look at the Alexander Technique:

Mental-Body Coordination:

Mindful Awareness: It entails becoming aware of and altering habitual movement patterns that generate strain or stress.

Movement Re-Education: Retrains the body to move with better comfort and efficiency.

Guide for somatic therapy

Alexander Technique Principles:
Primary Control: Highlights the link between the head, neck, and back, taking into account how this alignment affects general movement and posture.

Inhibition and Direction: Pauses and refrains from habitual reflexes or motions, followed by conscious directives for improved movement.

Core concepts:
Use of Self: Encourages people to think about how they use their bodies in daily tasks including sitting, standing, and walking.
Expansion and Release: Encourages the body to expand and move more easily by releasing unneeded tension.

Hands-on guidance and Feedback:
Gentle Touch: Instructors use gentle hands-on instruction to assist participants in

Guide for somatic therapy

recognizing and releasing tension, as well as improving body alignment.

Verbal Guidance: The use of verbal signals and commands to stimulate movement and postural modifications.

Applications in Everyday Life

Posture Improvement: Assists people in improving their posture and alignment whether sitting, standing, or doing other tasks.

Pain Reduction: This technique is frequently used to treat musculoskeletal pain, tension, and stress-related disorders by targeting movement patterns that cause discomfort.

The Alexander Technique has the following advantages:

Body Awareness:Encourages a better knowledge of how movement and posture impact general well-being.

Guide for somatic therapy

Improved Movement Efficiency: Aids in the performance of daily chores with less effort and stress, hence minimizing strain on the body.

Stress Reduction: Promotes relaxation and serenity by addressing and releasing unwanted bodily tension.

Incorporation into Daily Activities:

Applicable in a Variety of Settings: Individuals can incorporate the approach into a variety of activities, such as work, athletics, musical instrument playing, and so on.

Long-Term Learning: Learning the Alexander Technique necessitates continuing practice and application in daily life in order to effect long-term improvements in movement patterns.

The Alexander Technique promotes attention and conscious control over the body's motions, providing a practical way to

Guide for somatic therapy

improve movement and posture. Individuals may learn to move more effectively, minimize strain, and improve general well-being in their everyday lives with hands-on supervision, verbal prompts, and an emphasis on self-awareness. Individual classes with a licensed instructor are frequently used to teach it, with specific direction adapted to each individual's demands and movement patterns.

4. **Hanna Somatics movement :**

It is a method established by Thomas Hanna that focuses on re-educating the body and mind in order to alleviate chronic muscular tension and reestablish voluntary control over muscles. It incorporates movement, sensory awareness, and neuromuscular retraining. Here's a more in-depth look of Hanna Somatic Movement:

Pandiculation:

Controlled Movements: Hanna Somatics employs a method known as pandiculation, which is intentionally tightening and gently releasing muscles in order to reset and restore their normal length and function.

Re-Educating Muscles: This technique trains the brain to recover control of muscles that have become habitually clenched as a result of stress, injury, or repetitive actions.

Integration of Sensory and Motor Functions:

Mind-Body Connection: Highlights the relationship between sensory perception and movement, utilizing mindfulness to restore optimal muscular function.

Reprogramming Sensory Feedback: Individuals can restore voluntary control and lessen involuntary muscle contractions by reprogramming the sensory feedback loop.

Guide for somatic therapy

Three-Step Process:
Contract-Release-Re-educate: Individuals contract a muscle or muscle group intentionally, then gently release it while focusing on relaxation, before re-educating the brain for enhanced movement and muscular control.
Attention Promotion: Encourages attention and awareness of physical sensations during movement.

Emphasis on somatic Awareness :
Sensory-Motor Amnesia:Treats "sensory-motor amnesia," a condition in which the brain forgets how to relax particular muscles as a result of regular tension or stress.

Restoring Functional Movement: Promotes awareness of habitual patterns

Guide for somatic therapy

and facilitates conscious adjustment in order to restore functional movement.

Applications and Advantages:

Pain Relief: Used to treat chronic pain, muscle tension, and discomfort by resolving underlying muscular holding and tension patterns.

Improving Flexibility and Movement: By relieving chronic muscle contraction, it aids in enhancing flexibility, restoring natural movement, and improving posture.

Practice that is gentle and self-directed:

Self-Care Techniques:Many Hanna Somatic activities, such as gentle movements and self-directed pandiculation, may be done at home.

Educational Approach: Enables individuals to take an active role in their healing process by individually learning and implementing somatic movement practices.

Guide for somatic therapy

A Holistic Approach:

Mind-Body Integration: Recognizes the interdependence of mental and physical components, with a focus on restoring balance and well-being via somatic awareness.

Through the combination of sensory awareness and gentle, regulated movements.

Hanna Somatic Movement provides a comprehensive approach to relieving chronic muscle tension, optimizing movement patterns, and boosting general well-being. Individuals may decrease pain, enhance flexibility, and restore natural movement patterns by re-educating the brain to recover control over muscles, promoting a greater sense of ease and comfort in daily life. To encourage long-term improvements in muscle function and movement patterns, Hanna Somatic

Guide for somatic therapy

methods are frequently taught through a combination of practitioner-guided sessions and self-directed practice.

5.Trauma Releasing exercises:

Dr. David Berceli created Trauma Releasing Exercises (TRE) to release stress, tension, and trauma stored in the body through natural, spontaneous shaking or tremors. Here's some more information about TRE, along with several examples:

Relief of Stress and Trauma:

TRE focuses on stimulating the body's natural tremor or shaking mechanism, which allows the neurological system to release accumulated stress and tension.

The procedure is similar to animals' natural shaking reaction after a stressful experience, aiding the release of stored muscle tension.

Guide for somatic therapy

Tremors caused by oneself:
The exercises consist of a sequence of easy, self-guided motions and postures meant to cause modest muscular tremors or shaking.
For example, the practitioner may begin by resting on their back, elevating their legs, and gently pulsating or bouncing the knees to induce leg tremors.

Relaxation and release of muscles:
TRE seeks to relieve deep-seated muscle tension by letting the body tremble or shake spontaneously, encouraging relaxation and stress reduction.
As tremors arise throughout the exercises, individuals allow their bodies to shake or tremble without suppressing or regulating the action.

Process of Gradual Release:
At first, tremors may be modest and progressively built before diminishing gently,

Guide for somatic therapy

providing a sensation of relaxation and release.

As an example, shaking in one location may extend to other sections of the body, allowing for a complete release of stress.

Security and self-regulation:

During the process, TRE stresses the significance of safety and self-regulation, urging practitioners to respect their comfort level and boundaries.

For example, if the tremors become too powerful or overpowering, individuals are recommended to stop or adjust the exercises.

Integration and Grounding

Once the tremors have subsided, the exercises are frequently followed by grounding techniques such as deep

Guide for somatic therapy

breathing or soft movements to help restore a sense of peace.

For example, following the tremors, practitioners may switch to slow, deep breathing exercises or mild stretches to aid integration.

Use in Trauma Recovery:
TRE is used as a supplement in trauma recovery programs to aid in the release of accumulated stress and trauma from the body.
For example, therapists, counselors, and trauma survivors utilize it as part of a larger healing process to encourage relaxation and alleviate symptoms associated with trauma.

While TRE may give comfort for some, it is crucial to highlight that it is best practiced under the supervision of a qualified facilitator, especially for persons living with trauma or stress-related disorders. The goal of TRE is to give a natural, self-directed way

Guide for somatic therapy

for relieving tension and stress held in the body while also fostering relaxation and well-being.

6.Mindful Movement Techniques:

Mindful movement practices include a variety of strategies that integrate mindfulness with physical activity, encouraging a deeper mind-body connection and general well-being. Here's a primer on mindful movement techniques, complete with kinds, examples, and guidelines:

Mindful Movement Practices Come in a Variety of Forms:

a. **Yoga** is a practice that combines physical postures (asanas), breath control (pranayama), and meditation to improve flexibility, strength, and mental focus. Hatha, Vinyasa, and Restorative Yoga are a few examples.

Guide for somatic therapy

b. **Tai Chi** is an ancient Chinese martial practice that combines slow, flowing motions with deep breathing and meditation. It is intended to promote balance, flexibility, and inner tranquility.

c. **Qigong**: Like Tai Chi, Qigong uses gentle movements, synchronized breathing, and meditation to enhance the flow of energy (qi) throughout the body, increasing vigor and relaxation.

d. **Feldenkrais Method**: A technique that emphasizes awareness via movement, incorporating gentle and exploratory movements to enhance coordination, posture, and flexibility.

e. **Dance Meditation**:Using dance as a type of meditation to express oneself, release emotions, and develop bodily awareness via movement.

Guide for somatic therapy

Mindful Movement Practice Examples and Guidelines:

a. **Yoga:**

Examples: Sun Salutations (Surya Namaskar), Warrior Poses (Virabhadrasana), or Child's Pose (Balasana) practiced with concentrated breath awareness.

Guidelines:Concentrate on your breathing, move gently, and pay attention to your body's feelings. Avoid postures that are forced or strained, and exercise nonjudgmental awareness.

b. **Tai Chi**:

Examples: Tai Chi forms like "Grasp the Sparrow's Tail" or "Parting the Wild Horse's Mane."

Guidelines: Focus on gentle, flowing motions, synchronizing breath with movement, and maintaining calm, soft

Guide for somatic therapy

postures. Direct your attention within to detect minor changes in your body.

Qigong

Examples: Practicing "Five Animal Play" or "Eight Brocades" Qigong exercises.

Guidelines: While practicing the motions, focus on calm breathing, moving lightly and smoothly, and cultivating a sense of groundedness and relaxation.

Feldenkrais Method: Examples: Slow, exploratory motions such as rolling the head or pelvis, focusing on feeling and movement quality.

Guidelines: Slowly and attentively move your body, paying attention to sensations and tiny changes in movement. Instead of using force or strain, strive for ease and comfort.

Guide for somatic therapy

Dance Meditation:

Examples: Freestyle dancing while paying close attention to body motions, rhythm, and emotional expression.

Guidelines: Allow movement to emerge freely, focus on the feelings of dancing, and utilize it to express and release yourself.

Whatever practice is selected, the fundamental concepts are to cultivate mindfulness, focus on the present moment, and create a non-judgmental attitude toward oneself. Regularly practicing mindful movement can promote physical well-being, reduce stress, increase body awareness, and build a deeper connection between mind, body, and spirit.

Guide for somatic therapy

Mindful Movement:

Focused Attention:During yoga practice, attention is focused on body sensations, breath, and posture (asana) alignment.

Breath Awareness:Connecting breath and movement cultivates awareness of how the body responds and feels in various stances.

Body-Mind Connection: Exploration of Sensations: Yoga invites individuals to examine bodily sensations inside each pose, identifying tension, ease, resistance, or openness.

Observing Responses: Practitioners learn to notice emotional and physical reactions to different positions, allowing them to get a better awareness of their body-mind relationship.

Proprioception and Alignment:

Awareness of Body Positioning: Practicing yoga postures increases

Guide for somatic therapy

proprioception, which leads to greater alignment and postural awareness.

Focused Alignment: Paying attention to alignment signals increases awareness of how different motions or modifications influence comfort and stability.

Breath-Centered Practice: Conscious Breathing: Yoga stresses the use of the breath as a tool for somatic awareness, enabling practitioners to observe how breath impacts sensations and relaxation inside the body.

Breath Control: In yoga, breathwork methods (pranayama) assist control the neurological system, fostering calm and increased bodily awareness.

Mindfulness and Presence: Being Present: Yoga encourages practitioners to be completely present in their practice, allowing them to observe physical

Guide for somatic therapy

sensations, thoughts, and emotions without judgment.

Mindfulness Practice: Yoga helps individuals become more receptive to body experiences during practice by bringing attention to the present moment.

Mind-Body-Spirit Integration:
Holistic Approach: Yoga's holistic nature incorporates physical postures, breathwork, and meditation, allowing for a thorough investigation of the body-mind-spirit link.
Component Union: Yoga practice promotes body, mind, and spirit unification, allowing for a more integrated experience of somatic awareness.

Intention Setting:
Intentional Movement and Self-Exploration: Yoga practitioners are encouraged to make goals for their practice,

Guide for somatic therapy

focusing their attention on certain sensations, emotions, or parts of the body.
Self-Discovery: Individuals explore their limitations, sensations, and inner experiences via yoga, establishing a greater connection with their physical and emotional selves.

Yoga promotes somatic awareness by encouraging attentive movement, enhancing the body-mind connection, improving breath awareness, and building a deeper understanding of oneself. Regular yoga practice provides a transforming experience that increases general somatic awareness, resulting in enhanced physical, mental, and emotional well-being.

7.Mindful walking

Walking meditation, also known as mindful walking, is a practice that blends the physical exercise of walking with mindfulness practices. It entails paying

Guide for somatic therapy

close attention to feelings, motions, and surroundings while walking. Here are some more instances of attentive walking:

Sensory Awareness:
Foot Sensations: Notice the pressure, texture, and warmth of your feet when they make contact with the ground.
Body Movement: As you take each stride, be aware of the motions of your legs and body, feeling the muscles contract and relax.

Breath and Rhythm: Synchronized Breathing:Synchronize your breath with your steps by inhaling for a particular number of steps and expelling for the same number of steps, syncing your breath with the rhythm of your walk.
Natural speed: Walk at a comfortable speed, keeping a regular and steady rhythm and allowing for the natural flow of movement and breath.

Guide for somatic therapy

Watching surrounds:
Visual Awareness: Take in your surroundings by watching the colors, forms, and details without fixation, allowing your eyes to relax and take it all in.
Sound Awareness: Pay attention to the noises around you, whether they be the rustle of leaves, birds chirping, or distant traffic, and acknowledge each sound as it appears.

Mindful Intentions:
  Setting Intentions: Set an intention or focus for the exercise before beginning your walk, such as developing gratitude, finding serenity, or just being present in the moment.
Staying Present: If your mind wanders, softly restore your attention back to the present moment by gradually diverting your focus to the sensations of walking.

Guide for somatic therapy

Formal and Informal Practice: Dedicate specified time for a formal practice, strolling in a calm and uninterrupted environment, thoroughly immersing oneself in the attentive experience.

Everyday Mindful strolling: Integrate mindfulness into daily routines by practicing mindfulness throughout everyday walks, whether it's a stroll in nature, commuting, or strolling from one location to another.

Mindful Walking Practice Examples

Walking Meditation: As you walk in a specified area, take slow, deliberate steps, focusing on each movement, breath, and sensation.
Labyrinth Walking: Take a deliberate walk around a labyrinth, following the meandering path and focusing on the journey inner and outward.

Nature Walk: Take a walk in a natural area, such as a park or forest, paying attention to the sights, sounds, and fragrances of the environment while remaining careful of your surroundings.

Mindful walking allows individuals to improve present-moment awareness, alleviate stress, and connect more profoundly with themselves and their environment by putting mindfulness into motion. Mindful walking, whether done professionally or informally, may be a great technique for centering oneself and cultivating a sense of peace and clarity in daily life.

8. Dance movement therapy

Dance movement is a type of expressive movement in which physical movement is combined with emotional expression and self-exploration. Through movement, it

Guide for somatic therapy

helps people to connect with their bodies, emotions, and creativity. Here's more information about dance movement and how to practice it:

Dance Movement Forms

a.**Authentic Movement**: A practice that allows individuals to explore inner sensations and emotions via movement without the use of prescribed choreography.

b.**Ecstatic Dance**: An immersive, free-form dancing experience performed in a communal context that emphasizes self-expression, improvisation, and connection with the music and community.

c.**Dance/Movement Therapy**: A professional therapist uses dance and movement as a therapeutic therapy to treat emotional, physical, and psychological issues.

Guide for somatic therapy

d.**Conscious Dance**: Encourages conscious and deliberate movement via dance, with an emphasis on body awareness, self-exploration, and personal growth.

Dance Movement Practice:

a. **Create a Safe Space**:Identify a comfortable and secure setting in which you may move freely and without hesitation or judgment.

b.**Music Selection**: Select music that speaks to you or provokes feelings. It might be soothing, upbeat, rhythmic, or any other genre that promotes movement.

c.**Body Awareness and Warm-Up**: Begin with simple warm-up activities to get your body ready for activity.

Guide for somatic therapy

Close your eyes and check in with your body for a few seconds, recognizing any tightness or feelings.

d.**Exploration of Free Movement**: Begin moving your body in reaction to the music, allowing it to direct your motions.
-Be free to express yourself without regard for certain dance routines or technique.

e.**Emphasize Sensations**:Take note of how different motions feel in your body. As you move, pay attention to your sensations, emotions, and any energy shifts.

f. **Emotional Expression**:
Give yourself permission to express your feelings via movement. Dance may be used to help release emotions and tension.

g. **Mindful Presence**: Stay in the present moment, allowing your body to move instinctively. Engage in the event without judgment or self-criticism.

h.**Relaxation and Introspection**:
 Slow down your motions gradually, taking deep breaths to return to stillness.
-Take some time to contemplate or journal about any insights or feelings that came throughout the practice.

Benefits of dance movement
- Improves bodily awareness, expressiveness, and emotional release.
- Lowers tension, boosts mood, and promotes relaxation. Promotes creativity, self-confidence, and personal development.
- Promotes a sense of unity among the body, mind, and soul.

Individuals may tap into their intrinsic creativity, express emotions, and explore

Guide for somatic therapy

their inner world via the language of movement by engaging in dance movement activities. It is a liberating and therapeutic activity that promotes honesty, self-discovery, and overall health and well-being.

Guide for somatic therapy

Chapter 9 Integration and Transformation

Mind, Body, and Spirit Integration

Mind, body, and spirit integration is a holistic approach to well-being that emphasizes the connectivity and synergy between these components of human existence. Here's a more in-depth look at this integration:

1. **The Mind-Body-Spirit Connection:**

a. **Mind**: Thoughts, emotions, beliefs, perceptions, and cognitive processes all contribute to our experiences and actions.

Guide for somatic therapy

b. **Body**: The physical part of our life includes the concrete and material aspects of our existence, such as the body's structures, feelings, motions, and physiological activities.

C. **Spirit**: The spiritual part includes a feeling of purpose, meaning, values, a link to something larger, and the inner essence or awareness that exists beyond the physical sphere.

2. Holistic Approach to Happiness:

a. **Interdependence**: Accepts that the mind, body, and spirit are inextricably linked and impact each other's health and well-being.

b. **Harmony and Balance**:Strives for balance and harmony among these elements, realizing that disturbances in one may have an impact on the others.

Guide for somatic therapy

c. **Wholeness**: Aims for a sense of wholeness and integration by addressing health and wellbeing as a whole organism rather than discrete components.

3. **Integration Practices and Pathways**:

a. **Meditation and Mindfulness**:
Mindfulness techniques foster present-moment awareness by integrating the mind and body via focused attention and self-reflection.
 Meditation fosters a balanced link between mind, body, and spirit by promoting spiritual connection and inner calm.

b. **Holistic Healing Methods**:
Movement, breath, and mindfulness are used in yoga, tai chi, and qigong to link mind and body while also creating spiritual connections.
 Energy healing therapies such as Reiki and acupuncture try to balance the flow of

Guide for somatic therapy

energy inside the body, impacting mental, physical, and spiritual well-being.

c. **Creative Expression and Art Therapy**: Taking up art, music, dance, or other creative hobbies allows for self-expression while also assisting with emotional release and spiritual inquiry.

d.**Nature Connection and Grounding**: Spending time in nature ties people to the land and promotes a sense of grounding and spiritual connectivity.

4. Integration Advantages:

a.**Improved Well-Being**: Integration promotes a sense of completeness, which results in better mental, emotional, physical, and spiritual health.

Guide for somatic therapy

b.**Resilience and Coping**: Promotes adaptation and inner equilibrium by offering holistic tools for coping with life's obstacles.

c. **Inner Peace and Fulfillment**: Promotes inner peace, happiness, and a sense of purpose by facilitating a better awareness of oneself.

d.**Better Relationships**: A comprehensive approach to self-care fosters empathy, understanding, and compassion, which improves interpersonal interactions.

5. **Difficulties and Growth**:

a.**Inner Disconnection and Conflict**: Disconnection between mind, body, and spirit can result from conflicting ideas, trauma, or neglect, resulting in imbalance.

b.**Process of Healing and Integration**: Overcoming problems frequently entails a

Guide for somatic therapy

therapeutic process that includes the use of many techniques to reintegrate and regain equilibrium.

c.**Ongoing Journey**:Integration is a continual process that necessitates constant self-reflection, investigation, and adaptability to life's changes.

Mind, body, and spirit integration is a holistic approach to wellbeing that promotes harmony, balance, and connectivity among various elements of human existence. Individuals can enjoy significant well-being, resilience, and a greater feeling of purpose in life by embracing behaviors that foster this integration.

Guide for somatic therapy

Promoting long-term transformation

Somatic Therapy promotes long-term transformation by creating profound and long-lasting improvements in an individual's bodily, emotional, and psychological well-being. Here is a thorough examination of techniques of facilitating long-term transformation:

1.Understanding the Procedure:

a.**Somatic Awareness**: Encourages people to become more aware of their bodily feelings, emotions, and physical responses, allowing them to get a better knowledge of their internal experiences.

b.**Mind-Body Relationship**: Recognizes the interaction of ideas, emotions, and bodily experiences, highlighting their interdependence and influence on total well-being.

2 Holistic Healing and Integration:

a.**Addressing Root reasons**: Investigates and addresses the underlying reasons of discomfort, trauma, or pain held in the body, rather than just treating symptoms.

b.**Experience Integration**: Promotes the integration of fragmented or disowned components of oneself, producing a more coherent sense of self and a holistic healing process.

Guide for somatic therapy

3.**Therapeutic Modalities and Techniques**:

a.**Trauma-Informed Approaches**: Uses trauma-informed strategies to establish a safe atmosphere while respecting an individual's recovery pace and limits.

b. **Somatic Experiencing**: Uses physical sensations and movements to release stored trauma, enabling nervous system control and traumatic experience resolution.

c.**Therapies Focused on the Body**: Body-centered treatments such as yoga, dance therapy, or mindfulness-based activities are used to increase body awareness and relieve stress.

4.**Embodied Practices for Longevity**:

a.**Mindfulness and Self-Compassion**: Encourages mindfulness practice in order to

Guide for somatic therapy

be present with one's experiences and self-compassion in order to help the healing path.

b.**Resilience Building**: Emphasizes resilience building through somatic activities, the promotion of adaptive coping techniques, and the improvement of the capacity to deal with stresses.

c.**Empowerment and Self-Empathy**: Encourages people to create a sense of empowerment, self-agency, and self-empathy while going through the healing process.

5. Application in Daily Life:

a. **Continuous Learning and Practice**: Emphasizes that somatic healing is a continuous process, encouraging people to apply skills and concepts learnt in therapy in their daily lives.

Guide for somatic therapy

b. **Healthy Lifestyle Integration**: Incorporates somatic practices into everyday routines, encouraging healthy behaviors including activity, diet, appropriate sleep, and stress management.

6. Long-Term Support and Upkeep:

a.**continuous assistance**: Provides continuous assistance to maintain development and growth through frequent therapy sessions, group work, workshops, or community participation.

b.**Preventative and Self-Care Practices**: Encourages the use of self-care routines and practices that promote long-term well-being and help to avoid relapse or regression.

7.Personal Empowerment and Agency:

Guide for somatic therapy

a.**Client Empowerment**:Encourages clients to participate actively in their recovery path, generating a sense of empowerment, autonomy, and self-directed progress.

b.**Cultivating Resources**: Assists individuals in identifying internal and external resources that promote resilience and long-term transformation.

 Promoting long-term change through Somatic Therapy entails a multifaceted approach that addresses the mind-body connection, trauma-informed practices, embodied healing, resilience building, integration into daily life, ongoing support, and empowering individuals to be active participants in their healing journey. This complete method strives to establish long-term, deep-rooted changes that promote well-being and progress.

Guide for somatic therapy

Conclusion

We have gone on a profound journey by crossing the complicated and interwoven paths of Somatic Therapy, digging into the depths of our being in search of insight, healing, and profound transformation. This journey has been an examination, a discovery of the complicated interaction of our mind, body, and spirit, a journey that goes beyond just comprehending our physical and emotional sensations.

We've traveled the intricate landscapes of our feelings, decoded the histories contained within our physical form, and uncovered the deep knowledge embodied in our body's responses across these pages. Somatic Therapy has been a beacon of light, casting light on the deep interplay between our inner experiences, guiding us

Guide for somatic therapy

toward self-compassion, and maintaining an unbreakable connection to our real selves.

We've faced echoes of trauma, shadows lurking inside, and learnt the language of healing via the gentle embrace of Somatic Therapy embracing vulnerability, releasing stored tensions, and finding refuge in the safe havens we construct within ourselves.

This journey isn't only about comprehension; it's also a call to action, a celebration of perseverance, empowerment, and self-empathy. It is about embracing our vulnerabilities and finding strength in that vulnerability. It's about developing a garden of personal development and profound transformation by nourishing the seeds of self-awareness, compassion, and empowerment that lie dormant inside.

Somatic Therapy goes beyond the scope of these chapters and into the fundamental

Guide for somatic therapy

fabric of our being. Our days are shaped by the aware breaths we take, the attentive actions we do, and the empathic spaces we build inside ourselves. It's a never-ending invitation as a journey that weaves resilience, honesty, and self-awareness into the fabric of our existence.

As we close this chapter, let us carry the wisdom gained from these insights forward, cultivating a culture of understanding, empathy, and resilience within ourselves and our communities. May these lessons serve as beacons, illuminating our paths to comprehensive well-being, long-term development, and a greater connection to the symphony of life inside and around us.

This journey through Somatic Therapy demonstrates our ability for growth, tenacity in the face of adversity, and unshakable dedication to living truthfully. Let us embrace this insight, fostering it as a beacon of hope,

Guide for somatic therapy

directing us to a life rich in self-compassion, empowerment, and an unwavering connection to the dynamic core of our being.

Guide for somatic therapy

ABOUT THE AUTHOR

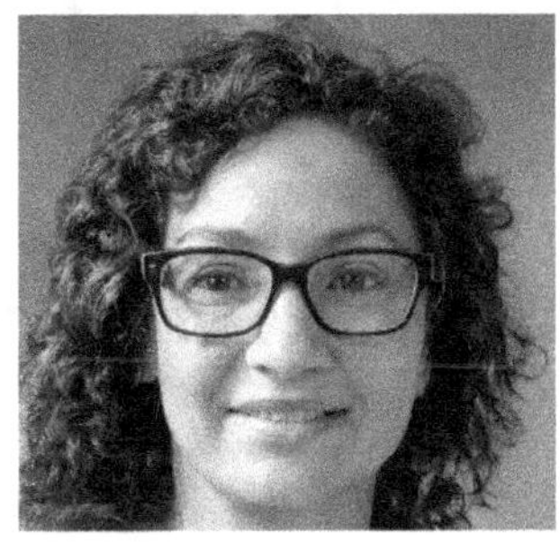

Dr. Elea Vandez is an impassioned advocate for the transformative power of healing, deeply committed to exploring and sharing the profound impact of somatic therapy in fostering holistic well-being. With a Doctorate in Psychology specializing in Somatic Therapy, she has dedicated her career to unraveling the intricate connections between mind, body, and spirit.

Driven by a fervent enthusiasm for the idea of healing, Dr Elea Vandez embarked on a journey of discovery, immersing herself in the realms of somatic awareness, trauma healing, and mindfulness practices. Her fervor and dedication have led her to

Guide for somatic therapy

become a sought-after speaker, educator, and practitioner in the field of mind-body healing.

Drawing from extensive clinical experience and a compassionate approach, she intertwines academic expertise with a profound understanding of human experiences. Her commitment to empowering individuals on their healing paths resonates through her teachings, publications, and workshops, emphasizing resilience, self-compassion, and the profound connection between internal and external well-being. Dr Elea Vandez passionately believes in the transformative potential within each individual, aiming to ignite a spark of self-awareness and empowerment through her work. Her boundless enthusiasm for the idea of healing infuses her writing with a warmth that resonates, inviting readers on a

Guide for somatic therapy

transformative journey toward holistic wellness and enduring self-discovery.

This book stands as a testament to Elea Vandez unwavering dedication to guiding others towards a life of authenticity, resilience, and profound healing, a journey she ardently hopes will inspire and empower readers to embrace the transformative power within themselves.

Guide for somatic therapy